Year-Around Conditioning for Part-Time Golfers

Books by Keith Jennison

Fiction

THE GREEN PLACE

For Children

FROM THIS TO THAT

Nonfiction

VERMONT IS WHERE YOU FIND IT
THE MAINE IDEA
DEDICATION
NEW HAMPSHIRE
NEW YORK AND THE STATE IT'S IN
GREEN MOUNTAINS AND ROCK RIBS
THE HALF-OPEN ROAD
THE BOYS AND THEIR MOTHER
THE AMERICAN INDIAN WARS (WITH JOHN TEBBEL)
REMEMBER MAINE
THE HUMOROUS MR. LINCOLN
YUP . . . NOPE AND OTHER VERMONT DIALOGUES
YEAR-AROUND CONDITIONING FOR PART-TIME
   GOLFERS (WITH DR. WILLIAM A. PRATT)

Editor

THE ESSENTIAL LINCOLN
THE CONCISE ENCYCLOPEDIA OF SPORTS

Year-Around Conditioning for Part-Time Golfers

How to Feel and Play Your Best All Your Life

William A. Pratt, M.D.,
and
Keith Jennison

Illustrated by Jim McQueen

Atheneum / SMI   1979   New York

DEDICATION

This book is dedicated, with respect and admiration, to all who have decided, or who will decide, that attaining physical fitness is not only the first answer to the challenge of playing better golf, but also the key to a longer and more vigorous life in which to enjoy this greatest of all games to the fullest.

Library of Congress Cataloging in Publication Data

Pratt, William Arthur, 1920–
    Year-around conditioning for part-time golfers.
    1. Physical fitness.   2. Golf.
I. Jennison, Keith Warren, joint author.
II. Title.
GV481.P76   613.7   78-53836
ISBN 0-689-10875-3

Copyright © 1979 by Keith Jennison
All rights reserved
Published simultaneously in Canada by McClelland and Stewart Ltd.
Composition by Connecticut Printers, Inc., Hartford, Connecticut
Printed and bound by Fairfield Graphics,
    Fairfield, Pennsylvania
Designed by Kathleen Carey
First Edition

Contents

	Introduction	3
1	What Is Fitness?	5
2	Fitness and Age	9
3	The Simplest Exercise of All	12
4	Before You Begin the Program	16
5	The Warm-ups	20
6	The Isotonic Exercises	28
7	Some Helpful Yoga Techniques	43
8	About Your Heart and Your Health Generally	46
9	The Aerobic Exercises	53
10	Aquadynamics	60
11	The Isometric Exercises	69
12	Some Specific Golfing Exercises	76
13	Your Weight and What to Do About It	82
14	Some Pointers to Playing Better	93
	USE YOUR POWERS OF VISUALIZATION	94
	HOLDING THE CLUB	97
	AIMING	100

CONTENTS

YOU DON'T NEED FORCE TO HIT A GOLF BALL	101
TAKE A LESSON NOW AND THEN	101
SWINGING RHYTHMICALLY	102
PRACTICING	103
STAYING LOOSE AND HAVING FUN	107
SOME WORDS FOR THE WISE	109
Weight Control Calorie Counter	111

Year-Around Conditioning for Part-time Golfers

Introduction

FOR MILLIONS OF PEOPLE of all ages, all over the world, there are few things in life quite as satisfying as a solidly struck golf shot. The rhythm of the swing, the crisp smack of the hit and the sight of the white ball arching above a green fairway against a blue sky fill the mind and heart with delight.

All the senses are involved in this experience. It is totally personal, and yet we seem to be at our best in the comradeship of golf. Perhaps that is because it is a game in which we and our opponents share mutual antagonists—ourselves and the golf course—and because the game makes strict demands on self-control and behavior, as well as on technical skills.

For many people, golf is simply a pleasant form of outdoor recreation. Relatively noncombative by na-

INTRODUCTION

ture, they accept the ups and downs of the game with equanimity and grace. They enjoy both being good companions and having them. It may be that these people get the most out of golf—mentally and physically. We hope that this book, and the conditioning program it suggests, will help them enjoy the game more and for a longer period of time.

Other golfers are high-strung, nervous perfectionists at heart. They respond to a topped drive, a shanked iron or a lipped putt with an explosion of anger and frustration.

Maybe golfers who have this reaction to imperfect shots would be better off considering some other, less frustrating form of recreation. But before they do, perhaps this book will help them play better enough to relieve the destructive reactions. We hope so.

Clearly, the more good shots you play, the lower your score will be and the better you will feel. Remember the first time you broke 100? Or 90? Or 80? How about your first subpar round?

Playing one's best golf, no matter what that best is, can be a goal for some and a dream for others. This is a book for people who love to play golf and want to play it as well as they can for the rest of their lives. It is a book about the reality of playing better golf, not the fantasy. But getting pars and birdies is not the whole story.

An elderly caddy at St. Andrews put it this way in commenting on a visitor whose clubs he carried. "He's nae much of a player, but he's a grand gowfer."

1: What Is Fitness?

I AM A VERMONT DOCTOR who started golfing late, but became increasingly devoted to this sometimes exhilarating and rewarding, sometimes depressing and frustrating game. As a golf addict myself, and as a doctor who treats other golf addicts, I have come to some opinions over the years as to how to play the game better and enjoy it more.

The golf season in Vermont is a short one, and I soon found out that if I didn't stay in shape year 'round, I got pretty frustrated with my summer golf game. So I joined the ranks of my fellow physical activists because it was evident that if one couldn't play golf to get fit, one could get fit to play better golf.

The point is well illustrated in the following table,

CHAPTER 1

which shows where golf ranks in physical fitness value.

It is a sad fact that many Americans can't pass a basic fitness test. We'll be talking a good deal about physical fitness in the following pages, so let's see how clearly we can define what we're talking about.

In a technical sense, physical fitness can be viewed as a measure of the body's strength, stamina and flexibility. In more meaningful personal terms, it is a reflection of your ability to work with vigor and pleasure, without undue fatigue, with energy left for enjoying hobbies and recreational activities, and for meeting unforeseen emergencies. It relates to how you look and feel, and because the body is not a compartment separate from the mind, it relates to your mental attitude as well as how you feel physically.

Physical fitness is many-faceted. Basic to it are proper nutrition, adequate rest and relaxation, sound health habits and good medical and dental care.

But these are not enough. An essential element is physical activity—exercise for a body that needs it to become and stay healthy.

Muscles make possible every overt motion. They also push food along the digestive tract, suck air into the lungs, tighten blood vessels to raise blood pressure when you need more pressure to meet an emergency. The heart itself is a muscular pump.

Technological advances have changed our way of living, making strenuous physical exertion largely unnecessary for most people, but the overall needs of the human body have not changed. Muscles are

Ratings were made on the basis of regular (minimum of four times per week), vigorous (duration of 30 minutes to one hour per session) participation in each activity.

	Jogging	Bicycling	Swimming	Skating (Ice or Roller)	Handball/Squash	Skiing-Nordic	Skiing-Alpine	Basketball	Tennis	Calisthenics	Walking	Golf*	Softball	Bowling
Physical fitness														
Cardiorespiratory endurance (stamina)	21	19	21	18	19	19	16	19	16	10	13	8	6	5
Muscular endurance	20	18	20	17	18	19	18	17	16	13	14	8	8	5
Muscular strength	17	16	14	15	15	15	15	15	14	16	11	9	7	5
Flexibility	9	9	15	13	16	14	14	13	14	19	7	8	9	7
Balance	17	18	12	20	17	16	21	16	16	15	8	8	7	6
General well-being														
Weight control	21	20	15	17	19	17	15	19	16	12	13	6	7	5
Muscle definition	14	15	14	14	11	12	14	13	13	18	11	6	5	5
Digestion	13	12	13	11	13	12	9	10	12	11	11	7	8	7
Sleep	16	15	16	15	12	15	12	12	11	12	14	6	7	6
Total	148	142	140	140	140	139	134	134	128	126	102	66*	64	51

*Ratings for golf are based on the fact that many Americans use a golf cart and/or caddy. If you walk the links, the physical fitness value moves up appreciably.

CHAPTER 1

meant to be used. When they are not, or not used enough, they deteriorate. If we are habitually inactive, if we succumb to the philosophy of easy living, we must then pay the price in decreased efficiency.

That we are, to a great degree, what our muscles make us—weak or strong, vigorous or lethargic—is a growing conviction among medical men.

More and more Americans are accepting the concept of a better and longer life through a program of physical conditioning. A great deal of credit for this awareness must be given to the splendid work of the President's Council on Physical Fitness, which was developed by John F. Kennedy from an existing program for youth fitness.

2: Fitness and Age

TOO MANY PEOPLE seem to feel that real physical fitness is possible only for the young. This is far from the truth.

You can't do much about getting older—you started the process the day you were born and you'll keep getting older as long as you live. But there are many misconceptions and unfortunate social attitudes that affect a person's outlook on aging, which is, after all, mostly a matter of the passing of time. For example, I have observed that many "older" people think that the physical problems they have, whether major or minor, are due simply to the fact that they are growing older.

I cannot say the following too strongly. *There are no symptoms, no complaints, no pains, no inability to do this or*

CHAPTER 2

that or the other, that can be attributed solely to the aging process. Show me a disease in a seventy-year-old and I can show you the same disease in a child.

One would be foolish to ignore the fact that, as the years go by, some of the full components of strength and energy are lost. But a substantial part of the reason for this is that people tend to conduct their lives differently as they get older. They are not as active as they used to be, and frequently they slow down just because they think they are *supposed* to slow down.

One elderly Vermonter who spent most of his time in a rocking chair was asked why he quit working. He said, "Pushing eighty is all the exercise I need." The figures in the following heart-disease mortality-rate table would seem to prove him wrong:

	CORONARY HEART DISEASE MORTALITY RATE FOR MALES			
AGE GROUP	*No exercise*	*Slight exercise*	*Moderate exercise*	*Heavy exercise*
40–49 years	238	179	162	132
50–59 years	506	484	426	385
60–69 years	1,490	1,177	856	682
70–79 years	3,307	2,470	1,803	1,161

Mortality rate for coronary heart disease decreased with increasing physical activity in each age group in a study of over 800,000 men and women from forty to seventy-nine years of age with no prior history of heart disease.

The danger in accepting a disability or dysfunction of the body as just part of "getting older" lies in not finding out specifically what is causing it. Over and over again I have seen physical conditions identified, treated and relieved that the aging patient had viewed, like death and taxes, as inevitable.

Golfers in their middle years would do well to consider the career of Gene Sarazen. Gene won the U.S. Open in 1922 when he was twenty years old. He won the PGA the same year, won it again the following year, and again ten years later. He took the British Open in 1932 and the Masters in 1935 with a double eagle that just may be the greatest pressure shot ever played in tournament golf. Gene, at seventy-six, still plays or practices almost every day and scores his age.

There is absolutely no reason why you shouldn't strive for a similar goal.

3: The Simplest Exercise of All

IF YOU ARE ONE of the millions of Americans who have already embarked on a physical-conditioning program, you are well aware of the results—the feeling of well-being and an improved self-image. If you have not yet taken up such a program, we urge you to do so. A sound, faithfully followed fitness program has changed countless lives for the better.

The program we recommend in this book is specifically aimed at improving your golf game, but it should be evident that the specific golf exercises won't accomplish this unless the whole body is conditioned and toned. Of course, we place special emphasis on the body movements that are most directly involved in playing golf, but if you are going to play the best golf you are capable of, you shouldn't limit your exercise schedule to special golf routines.

If you are currently under a doctor's care, you would do well to discuss the matter of an exercise program with him. Most people are potentially in much better shape than they think they are, but there is always a chance that a doctor who knows your medical problems, if you have any, might want to make some adjustments in the program you have chosen. If you haven't had a complete physical examination for a year or so, it might be a good idea to have a checkup. If you think that age is slowing you down, you'll probably find that this isn't the case at all. What you really need is exercise.

Let's start with the simplest exercise there is. No matter what kind of golf you play now, or if you're just beginning, there's one thing you can do as well as any professional on the circuit. You can *walk*. You can walk, not ride, the golf course. Of course, the touring pros *have* to, and you don't, but the more walking you do, both off and on the course, the better will be both your golf and your health.

As you walk, think about the *way* you do it. Do you walk tall with your head and chest held high? If you don't, start walking that way now and never walk any other way. Swing your legs forward from the hip joints, keeping the knees and ankles limber. Push your feet off the ground, don't shuffle. Walk as if you owned the golf course—you probably don't, but at least you're renting it. Walking between shots keeps

THE SIMPLEST EXERCISE OF ALL

CHAPTER 3 the body warm and the muscles limber. Sitting in a cart doesn't.

Depending on how much criss-crossing you do from rough to rough, if you're off your game, you may walk four miles or more during an 18-hole round. Stay out of motorized carts as much as you can. Take a caddy or pull your clubs on a cart. If you have to take a cart when playing in a foursome, take one cart instead of two and trade off if you get tired.

While walking to your next shot, concentrate on exactly where you want it to go and *visualize* it going there. After holing a fairway wood for a 2 on a par-5 hole in the 1935 Masters, Gene Sarazen is reported to have said, "Where did you think I was aiming?"

Some years back I played the Rutland Country Club course many times with Bobby Locke. He walked, of course, and, more than that, he tried to keep everything at the same pace. He walked deliberately, addressed the ball slowly and then made his shot. On the green, he always took a couple of practice swings with the putter, set his stance and putted. Whenever I played with him, I observed that his rhythm never changed—not only the speed of his swing but of every movement he made during the whole round.

I remember Locke as a delightful man and a splendid golfer. Just a little while ago, I read a report of the first round of the 1977 Hall of Fame Golf Classic at the famous (or infamous to some golfers) No. 2 Course at the Pinehurst Country Club. Bobby had been inducted into the World Golf Hall of Fame two

THE SIMPLEST EXERCISE OF ALL

days before. Locke is sixty now and doesn't play much tournament golf anymore. A reporter asked him about his round. "I'm striking the ball quite well," he said, "but just a bit more frequently than I used to."

Take it easy and relax. It is far better for you to take your time, walk and play nine holes than it is for you to rent a cart and race through 18. What counts is how many strokes it takes you to hole out—not how many minutes it takes you to play them.

If you swoop down the fairway in your cart, leap out of your seat and pounce on your ball like a hungry tiger, your chances of playing the shot well are considerably diminished.

4: Before You Begin the Program

THERE ARE MANY PROGRAMS for achieving physical fitness. Some of them go by names that may be familiar, yet meaningless, to you. To name a few: AEROBICS, ISOTONICS, ISOMETRICS, AQUADYNAMICS and YOGA. Each has benefits, but rarely do the proponents of any particular method concede the value of another.

Our simple conditioning program is based on a combination of these five exercise disciplines, so let's start by explaining them briefly.

AEROBICS are defined as exercises that stimulate, condition and improve heart, lung and vascular functions. The value of these exercises is in direct proportion to the length of time you devote to them. They develop stamina and agility.

BEFORE YOU BEGIN THE PROGRAM

ISOTONICS are the exercises of repetitive movement. These are systematically planned to tone and strengthen major muscle groups.

ISOMETRICS are exercises of no lineal movement at all. Muscles or muscle groups are pitted against other muscles or muscle groups or against immovable objects.

AQUADYNAMICS is a sophisticated word for exercises done in the water.

YOGA, having spiritual as well as physical implications, is hard to define. Basically, it is a system of held postures and relaxation rather than of movement.

The exercise program that follows is designed to improve both your golf game and your overall health. Take it seriously, but take it slowly and carefully at first. You may begin with all the enthusiasm of the recent convert and overdo some of the exercises involving muscles which have become weak and flabby from lack of use. Overdoing a specialized exercise might have a very adverse effect upon your golf game. Think about what happened to Jerry Pate, for instance.

Not long after he won the U.S. Open in 1976, Pate was reported "to have tried his strength twisting a muscle-building device and felt a pain in his shoulder." The pain persisted and increased in spite of everything doctors could do. Early in 1977, Pate won at Phoenix, but the pain got worse and he left the tour for two months of rest and therapy. In the 1977 U.S. Open at Southern Hills, he finished well down in the list.

CHAPTER 4

12-MINUTE TEST FOR MEN
(Distance in miles covered in 12 minutes)

	AGE			
FITNESS CATEGORY	Under 30	30–39	40–49	50+
I. Very Poor	< 1.0	< .95	< .85	< .80
II. Poor	1.0–1.24	.95–1.14	.85–1.04	.80– .99
III. Fair	1.25–1.49	1.15–1.39	1.05–1.29	1.0 –1.24
IV. Good	1.50–1.74	1.40–1.64	1.30–1.54	1.25–1.49
V. Excellent	1.75+	1.65+	1.55+	1.50+

< Means less than.

The exercise program we advocate requires no special equipment or clothing, and many of the exercises can be performed in your home, office or hotel room if you are on a trip. Some of them can be practiced even when you are driving a car, while others can be worked at during the commercials that interrupt your favorite TV show.

Pace yourself and don't expect miracles. If you take the program seriously, you will show quick and steady improvement. Your golf scores will go down, your enjoyment of the game will increase, and you'll feel better about a lot of other things besides your golf.

Before you even begin the program, you might like to find out what kind of shape you're in to start with.

Ten years ago, Dr. Kenneth Cooper published the first of several fine conditioning books based on aerobics, defined as that form of exercise which forces the body to consume increased amounts of oxygen. His books have sold in the millions and have

BEFORE YOU BEGIN THE PROGRAM

12-MINUTE TEST FOR WOMEN*
(Distance in miles covered in 12 minutes)

FITNESS CATEGORY	AGE			
	Under 30	30–39	40–49	50+
I. Very Poor	< .95	< .85	< .75	< .65
II. Poor	.95–1.14	.85–1.04	.75– .94	.65– .84
III. Fair	1.15–1.34	1.05–1.24	.95–1.14	.85–1.04
IV. Good	1.35–1.64	1.25–1.54	1.15–1.44	1.05–1.34
V. Excellent	1.65+	1.55+	1.45+	1.35+

*Preliminary chart based on limited data.
< Means less than.

made invaluable contributions to the dramatically increased commitment, on the part of many thousands of men and women, to exercise programs of walking, jogging, running, bicycling and swimming.

Through carefully designed and controlled testing methods, Dr. Cooper developed data of great value in assessing physical condition. His publishers, M. Evans and Company, have kindly given us permission to reprint his simple, basic physical-fitness test which anyone can try with a minimum of time and effort. All it involves is seeing how much level ground you can cover in 12 minutes. If you're not already a runner or jogger, walk a little first to warm up, then jog, then walk.

5: The Warm-ups

THERE ARE ALL KINDS of learning experiences. We learn something from every round of golf we play, perhaps not consciously, but the continuing effort to do something right is certain to have a beneficial effect.

Learning concentration is part of this exercise program. Even in the simple warm-up exercises, concentrate on doing them properly. Sloppily performed movements will do you some good, but nowhere nearly as much as if you keep your mind on precisely what you are trying to do.

These warm-up exercises have been carefully selected and should be done in the order listed. They will ventilate your lungs, warm up your heart and loosen major muscle areas.

If you can't spare the time for a full workout, do these anyway—any time, any place. For example, if you have been concentrating for a couple of hours at a desk, or on a long TV special, get up and do them. Your tension will be relieved and you'll feel relaxed and refreshed.

One result of doing the brief exercises several times a day is that people who do them forget to take tranquilizers.

This is a diagram of the square-to-line golfing stance. "Square" means that your body is set squarely on a line parallel to the visualized flight line of the ball.

Set your feet in this position for all exercises that are performed, standing erect without moving your feet. This will help integrate many body movements with your golf stance.

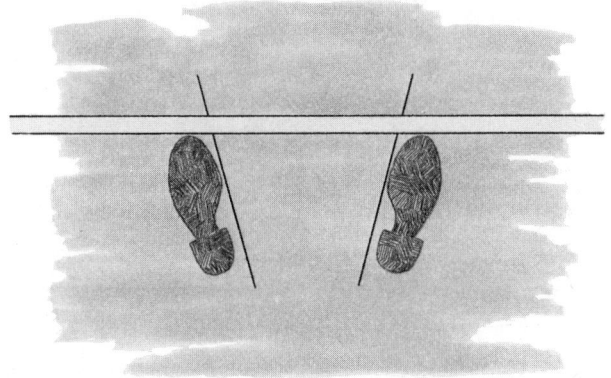

Now, a few words about breathing. One of the finest Yoga concentrations is abdominal breathing.

CHAPTER 5

Putting it another way, think about filling your stomach with air instead of your lungs. Stick out your stomach as you inhale and pull it back in as you let out your breath. In general, as you exercise, draw your breath in through your nose and let it out through your parted lips. Take a deep breath just before the first count of any exercise, exhale as the muscles contract in the exercise, and take another deep breath when returning to the starting position.

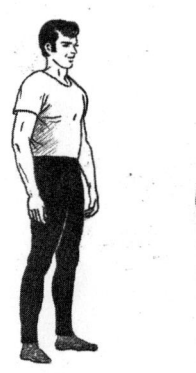
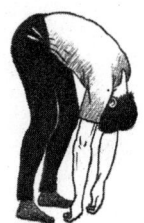

1. BEND AND STRETCH

Starting position: Feet in square-to-line golfing stance.
Action: Count 1—Bend trunk forward and

down, flexing knees. Stretch gently in attempt to touch fingers to toes or floor. Count 2—Return to starting position.
Repeat: Ten times.
Note: Do slowly, stretch and relax at intervals rather than in rhythm.

Remind yourself to breathe properly—start with a full, deep breath, exhale while bending down and inhale coming up. Take *deep* breaths. Don't strain to touch your toes. It's the reaching that matters, not the touching.

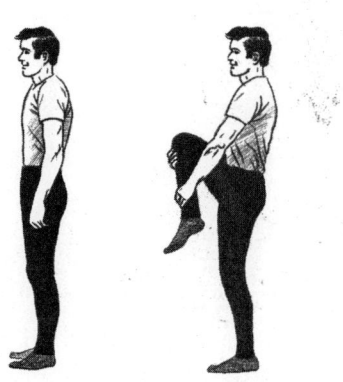

2. KNEE LIFT

Starting position: Stand erect, feet together, arms at sides.
Action: Count 1—Raise left knee as high as possible, grasping leg with hand and pulling knee against body while keeping back straight. Count 2—Lower to starting position. Repeat with right knee on counts 3 and 4.
Repeat: Ten right and ten left.

CHAPTER 5

This loosens up the big thigh muscles and also helps improve your sense of balance. You may stagger around a little the first few times you do this one, but don't let that bother you. And remember your breathing.

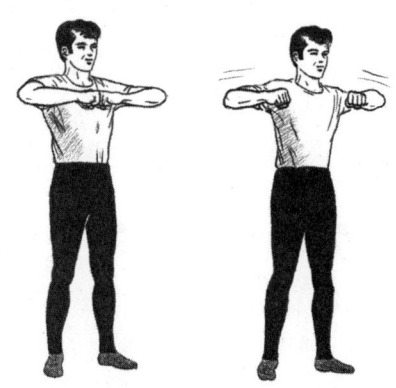

3. WING STRETCHER

Starting position: Stand erect, elbows at shoulder height, fists clenched in front of chest.
Action: Count 1—Thrust elbows backward vigorously without arching back. Keep head erect, elbows at shoulder height. Count 2—Return to starting position.
Repeat: 20 times.

Tones upper arm, neck and back muscles, which are all vital to your shotmaking.

THE WARM-UPS

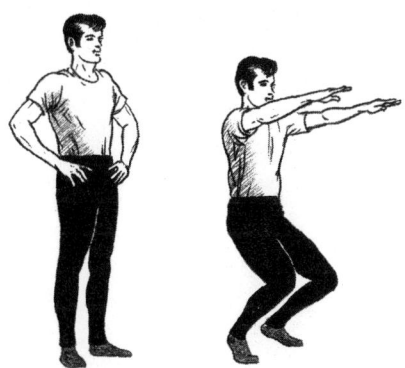

4. HALF KNEE BEND

Starting position: Stand erect, hands on hips.
Action: Count 1—Bend knees halfway while extending arms forward, palms down. Count 2—Return to starting position.
Repeat: 20 times.

This is more leg warm-up. Remember to raise your heels, which will help develop the proper foot action for the golf swing.

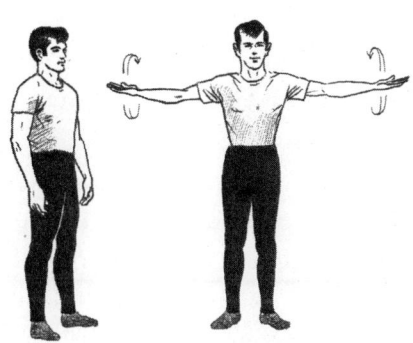

5. ARM CIRCLES

Starting position: Stand erect, arms outstretched sideward at shoulder height, palms up.
Action: Make small circles backward with

hands, keeping head erect. Do 15 backward circles. Reverse the action, turning palms down and making 15 circles forward.
Repeat: 15 times in both directions.

Again, this is an excellent way to develop the golfer's all-important upper-arm and shoulder muscles.

6. THE SHOULDER TURN

Note that at the top of the swing, illustrated on page 96, the shoulders have moved through a full 90 degrees and are now at a right angle to the line of the stance. This shoulder turn is vital to good shotmaking. Without it you will probably try to compensate by increased hand and arm action, thereby losing rhythm, power and accuracy.

How can you make this movement naturally and instinctively if you never turn your body in this exact way unless you are on the golf course? The answer is, you can't. It must be practiced.

Many manuals have an exercise called the body turn. This is customarily performed with the arms extended at shoulder level and calls for a rotating movement at the waist. It's a good exercise, but we can make it a far better one for your golf game by adding a few variations.

Start by placing your driver across your shoulders at the back of your neck, extending your arms fully and hooking them over the club. Take a few easy back and forth turns this way and see how good it feels. Here's the exercise in full:

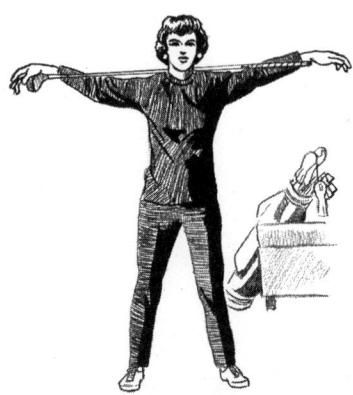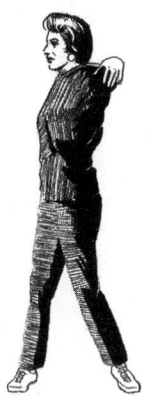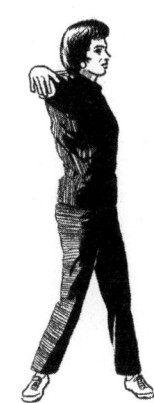

Starting position: Stand erect, feet in the golfing stance and eyes fixed on a particular spot on the wall in front of you.

Action: While keeping your head motionless, turn your shoulders and hips to the right until your shoulders face the wall on your right. As you make the turn, let your body weight transfer to your firm, but not locked, right leg. To accommodate this weight shift, your *left* heel will raise slightly. Repeat the exact movement turning to the left, letting your weight transfer smoothly to a firm left side and your *right* heel rising. Be sure not to sway, and be sure your head doesn't move.

Repeat: As many times as you can and as often as you can.

This exercise is especially good for warming up at the first tee.

6: The Isotonic Exercises

THE NEXT TWO GROUPS of exercises, the isotonics and the aerobics, have suggested graded attainment levels to help you keep track of your progress.

Let me remind you to *take it easy* when you start the program. Your body knows its capacity better than you do. The last thing we want is for you to feel so stiff and sore from doing exercises that you can't enjoy playing golf the next day.

Do not go from level C to level B until your body almost demands it. Many experts in the field have recorded a distressing number of dropouts among those who embark on a disciplined exercise program. There are various reasons for this, but the most frequent one appears to be the result of doing the exercises to excess early on in the program, resulting in pulled muscles, strained tendons, aching backs and general fatigue. Remember, you're not training for the Olympic decathlon, you're just investing a few hours a week in the present and future of your golf game—and your life.

Each exercise is accompanied by a repetition level guide. Depending on your physical condition, you will proceed from one level to the next at different rates. It would be better if you didn't mix the levels due to discovering that one exercise was easier to perform than another. Wait until you can perform *all* the exercises with equal facility before you move up.

When you first begin, take your time. Your goal, of course, is to complete the exercise group in as short a time as possible—but work up your speed *gradually*.

In the box marked "Start" in the repetition guide (see page 32), enter the number of times you do an exercise when you start the program. The page describing the last isotonic exercise has a box to record the total time spent in doing *all* the exercises, including the warm-ups. Keeping records is a fine way to prove to yourself the rewarding improvement in your physical capabilities.

THE ISOTONIC EXERCISES

THE PUSHUPS

We'll start this group of isotonic exercises with the familiar pushup. (Remember to do your warm-ups before you start.) The pushup is an important exercise for golfers in that it strengthens the upper-arm, shoulder and upper-back muscles, which are essential to good shotmaking. Research indicates that these muscles are among the first to deteriorate through being less involved in daily activity.

Three pushup exercise methods are illustrated. Begin with the first and, if that's too easy, go on to the second and eventually to the third.

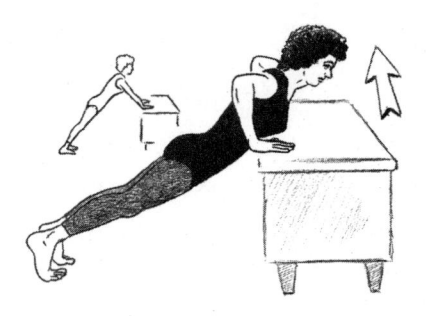

1.

Starting position: Lean with extended arms against the edge of a firm table, chest of drawers, dresser or bed end.
Action: Bend the arms slowly until the chest touches the hands, then extend the arms fully again. Keep breathing regularly.
Note: Your graduated repetition guide (page 32) is adjusted to the third method. Do not go on to the B level until you are doing the required number of repetitions of the third method.

THE ISOTONIC EXERCISES

2.

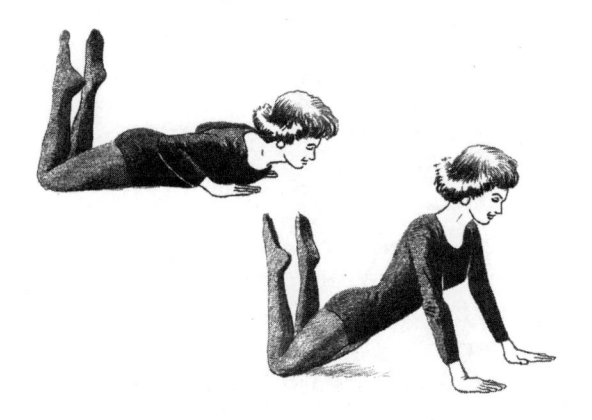

Starting position: Lie on floor, face down, with your legs together, knees bent with feet raised off the floor. Hands, palms down, are on floor under shoulders.
Action: Count 1—Push upper body off the floor until the arms are fully extended and the body is in a straight line from head to knees. Count 2—Return to starting position.

3.

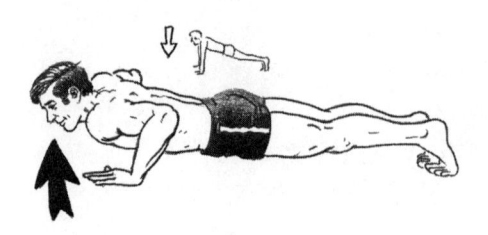

Starting position: Lie on the floor, face down, legs together. With fingers pointing straight ahead, the hands are on the floor under the shoulders.

Action: Count 1—Push body off the floor by extending arms, so that the weight rests on the hands and toes. Count 2—Lower the body until the chest touches the floor.

Note: Body should be kept straight, buttocks should not be raised, abdomen should not sag.

REPETITION LEVELS

Start	C	B	A
	4	10	15

THE ANKLE STRETCH

This exercise is designed to stretch and condition the Achilles tendons and the muscles of your calves. Before the coming of the horseless carriage, not too many people had trouble in this area. Children and most adults kept their lower leg muscles supple and strong by walking a lot. If you are going to play your best golf and have your body move in harmony, these muscles and tendons must be kept in shape. This

THE ISOTONIC EXERCISES

exercise is particularly important for women golfers. Depending on how many years they have been walking around on high heels, the length of their Achilles tendons may actually have shortened.

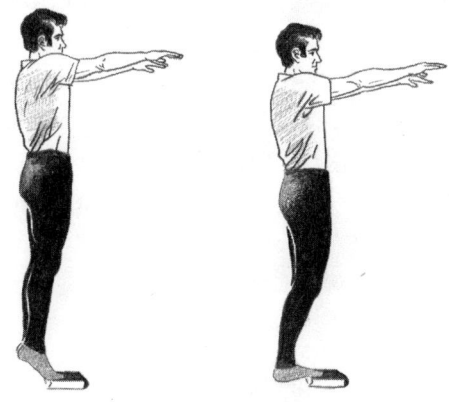

Starting position: Stand on a stair, large book or block of wood, with weight on the balls of the feet and the heels raised.
Action: Count 1—Lower heels. Count 2—Raise heels.

REPETITION LEVELS

Start	C	B	A
	10	20	30

THE SIT-UPS

Now we'll go to work on your abdominal muscles, which, if you are anything like most people, probably need it. Carrying around a front porch is bad for your back and worse for your golf game.

CHAPTER 6

The illustration below shows you how the exercise ultimately *should* be done, but you'll probably have to work for a number of weeks before you can manage it this way. Some manuals suggest that you start doing sit-ups with your feet tucked under something to hold them down while you raise your torso. The exercise is certainly easier this way, but the problem is that it's *too* easy. Many orthopedic doctors have patients who have lower back problems as a result of doing too many sit-ups this way too enthusiastically, too soon.

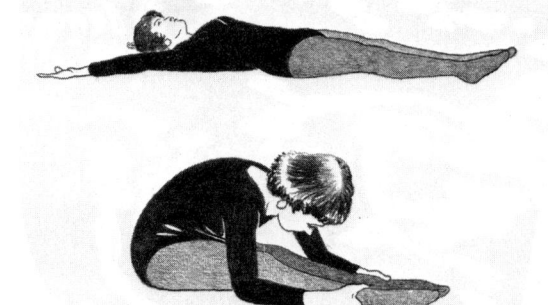

Starting position: Lie on back, legs straight and together, arms extended beyond head.
Action: Count 1—Bring arms forward over head, roll up to sitting position, sliding hands along legs, grasping ankles. Count 2—Roll back to starting position.

REPETITION LEVELS

Start	C	B	A
	10	15	20

Doing this exercise incorrectly at the beginning could keep you off the golf course for weeks. So we would prefer to have you start with some related exercises that will prepare you to do the sit-ups only when you are ready to. You might start with this one.

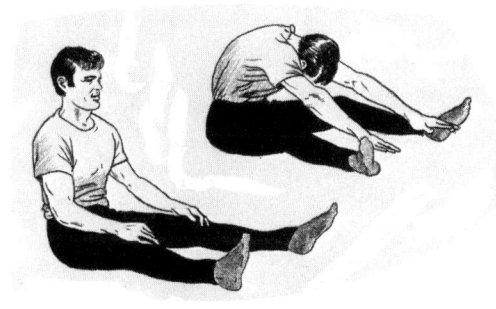

THE ISOTONIC EXERCISES

SITTING STRETCH

Starting position: Sit, legs spread apart, hands on knees.
Action: Count 1—Bend forward at waist, extending arms as far forward as possible. Count 2—Return to starting position.

And/or this one:

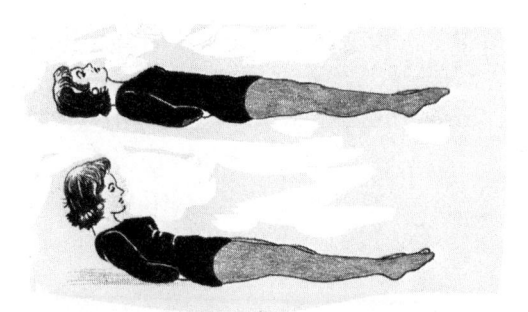

HEAD AND SHOULDER CURL

Starting position: Lie on back, hands tucked under small of back, palms down.
Action: Count 1—Tighten abdominal muscles, lift head and pull shoulders and elbows off floor. Hold for 4 seconds. Count 2—Return to starting position.

Of course, the following exercise, the leg-ups, will also help you get ready for the full sit-up exercises.

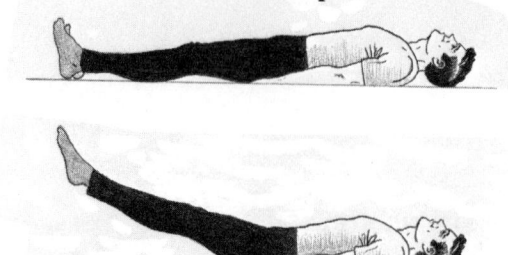

THE LEG-UPS

Starting position: Lie on back, legs straight and extended, hands palms down under buttocks. *Action:* Raise both legs about 18 inches with toes pointing forward. Lower slowly until heels just touch floor and repeat.

REPETITION LEVELS

Start	C	B	A
	10	20	25

The leg-ups concentrate on the lower muscles of the abdomen, while the sit-ups involve the upper abdominal muscles more directly.

Speaking of the abdominal muscles reminds me to comment on the question of what is the best time of day to exercise. I am inclined to recommend that you do these exercises first thing in the morning, although it is better to do them whenever you have the opportunity rather than not do them at all on any given day.

The classic phrase for these exercises, setting-up exercises, has real meaning in that they do set you up for the rest of the day. You can do them right after you get up and ease into the others later on in the morning or afternoon, depending on what kind of day you have.

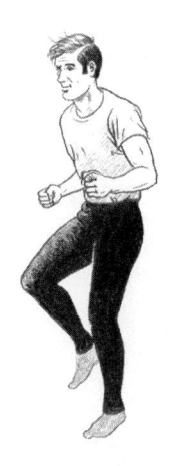

THE ISOTONIC EXERCISES

RUNNING IN PLACE

Run in place, raising each foot at least 4 inches off floor on each step. Count "one" each time left foot touches floor.

The way to do this is to start with 25 left-foot counts. Then do five straddle hops (see below). Then repeat the 25 running steps, then do five more straddle hops. Start with 2 minutes at the C level.

REPETITION LEVELS

Start	C	B	A
	2 min.	4 min.	6 min.

CHAPTER 6

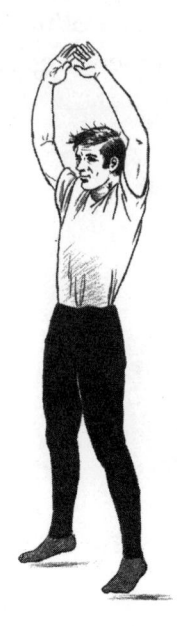

STRADDLE HOP

Starting position: Square-to-line golfing stance. *Action:* Count 1—Swing arms sideward and upward, touching hands above head (arms straight) while simultaneously moving feet sideward and apart in a single jumping motion. Count 2—Spring back to starting position.

REPETITION LEVELS

Start	C	B	A
	10	20	30

THE STEP TEST

You will, of course, be able to observe the increase in your strength and stamina—and your general feeling of well-being—from week to week in many ways, including the increasing facility with which you do the exercises.

In addition, there is a 2-minute step test you can use to measure and keep a continuing record of the improvement in your circulatory efficiency, one of the most important of all aspects of fitness.

The immediate response of the cardiovascular system to exercise differs markedly between well-conditioned individuals and others. The test measures the response in terms of pulse rate taken shortly after a series of steps up and down onto a bench or chair.

Although this test does not take long, it is necessarily vigorous. Stop if you become overly fatigued while taking it.

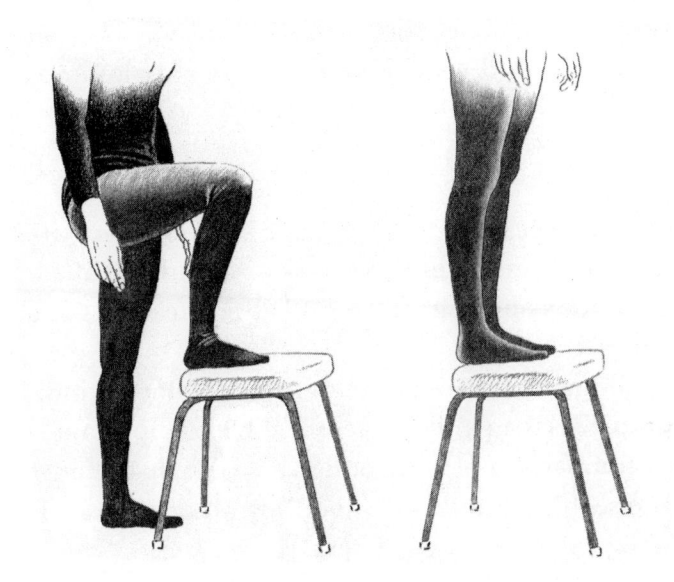

THE ISOTONIC EXERCISES

CHAPTER 6

The test: Use a sturdy bench or chair 15 to 17 inches in height.
Count 1—Place right foot on bench.
Count 2—Bring left foot alongside right foot and stand erect.
Count 3—Lower right foot to floor.
Count 4—Lower left foot to floor.

REPEAT the four-count movement 30 times a minute for 2 minutes.
THEN sit down on bench or chair for two minutes. FOLLOWING the 2-minute rest, take your pulse for 30 seconds. Double the count to get the per-minute rate. (You can find the pulse by applying middle and index finger of one hand firmly to inside of wrist of other hand, on the thumb side.)

Record your score for future comparisons. In succeeding tests—about once every two weeks—you probably will find your pulse rate becoming lower as your physical condition improves.

Three important points:

1. For best results, do not engage in physical activity for at least 10 minutes before taking the test. Take it at about the same time of day and always use the same bench or chair.

2. Remember that pulse rates vary among individuals. This is an individual test. What is important is not a comparison of your pulse rate with that of anybody else, but rather a record of how your own rate is reduced as your fitness increases.

3. As you progress, the rate at which your pulse is lowered should gradually level off. This is an indication that you are approaching peak fitness.

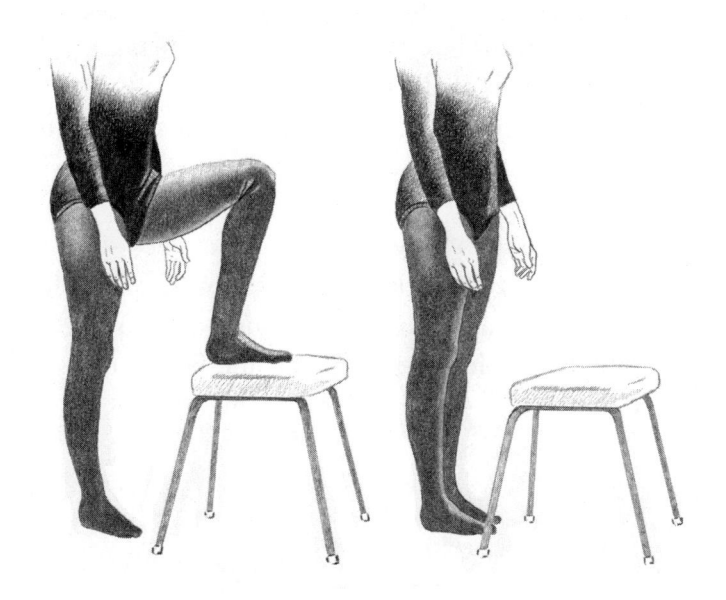

THE ISOTONIC EXERCISES

The new world of physical conditioning is full of well-advertised programs guaranteeing incredible results attained by devoting ten or so minutes a day to doing a few prescribed rudimentary exercises.

It isn't quite that simple. No two human bodies are the same, nor will they respond equally to the same routines.

This book puts the emphasis on doing the warm-ups once a day, then adding one or more exercise sessions chosen from the other groups—as time and circumstance permit.

Let's face it, the only exercise program that you are

CHAPTER 6 going to follow for any length of time is the one you make up for yourself because it makes you feel consistently better as the months go by. This book tells you all you need to know about creating a *personal* program that will change and develop as your unique body tells you what it needs and wants.

Many programs put great stress on the speed with which you can complete any particular group of exercises. So do we. However, speed in executing the isotonic exercises in no way replaces the necessity for following an aerobic schedule, because the aerobics develop stamina and endurance—just what you need for a tough 18-hole match which could be decided on the last hole.

7: Some Helpful Yoga Techniques

BEFORE WE GO to the aerobics, we would like to introduce you to some Yoga techniques that you may find relaxing and beneficial.

The objectives of Yoga are calmness and relief from tension and anxiety. To a great degree, then, the practice of this art or discipline is a mental one as well as a physical one. The effects of tension and anxiety are well known to all golfers—especially when there is a great deal at stake. The ability to direct your body to relax and your mind to clear itself of extraneous concerns *can* be developed, and you might do well to begin to acquire this ability.

For example, when you have finished a set of the warm-ups, try the Yoga posture of relaxation.

For a while you may be aware of a strong heartbeat. Don't worry about it—just listen to it and relax. Your

CHAPTER 7

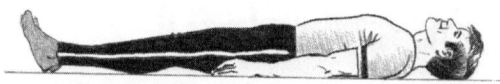

heart's doing just what it is supposed to be doing—adjusting to decreased demands from various parts of your body.

After a moment or so, "give orders" to your body to relax. Start with the feet, then go up the legs, the abdomen, the chest, arms, shoulders and back and, finally, into the mind itself.

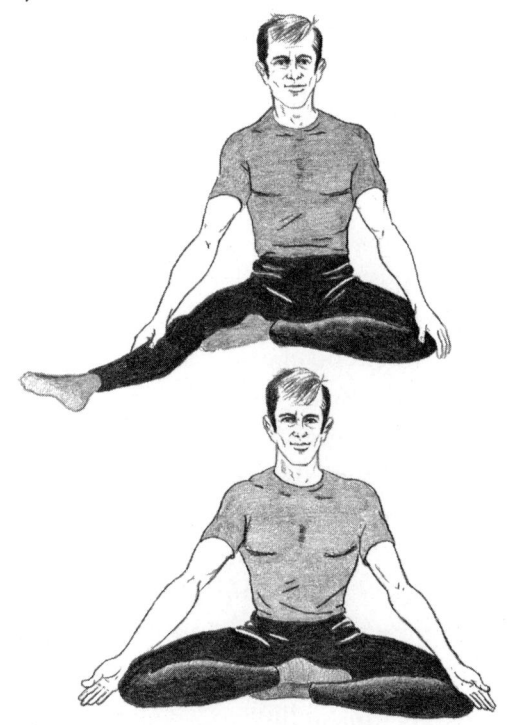

When you have completed this procedure, sit up and assume the traditional Yoga posture illustrated here. It is particularly well adapted for rest breaks in your exercises. Do some deep-breathing abdominal exercises and rerun your private videotape of the best shots you played during your last round of golf.

In case you don't know it, your circulatory system works something like a two-lane highway. Your heart pumps blood out through your arteries and brings it back through your veins. To one degree or another, gravity is a factor. That's one reason why lying down is more restful than standing up. The Yoga posture illustrated below changes the gravity factor, and Yoga enthusiasts, not without reason, claim many beneficial results.

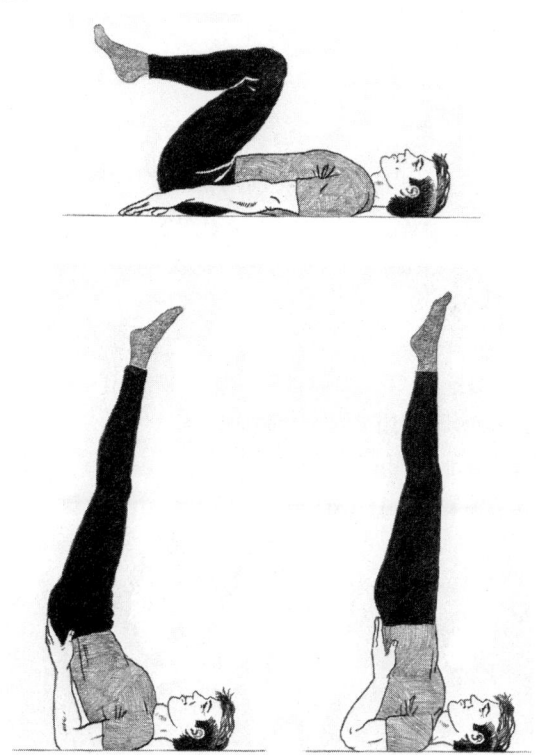

SOME HELPFUL YOGA TECHNIQUES

8: About Your Heart and Your Health Generally

AMERICAN MEN AND WOMEN are now living longer and more productive lives than ever before in our history. One of the reasons is clearly the increased knowledge the medical profession has about the prevention, early diagnosis and successful treatment of disease. The media have contributed greatly to increased public concern about national health problems, and many sporting events and volunteer agencies have contributed to the result with massive funding.

In the decade of the 1960's, life expectancy in the United States increased by only 0.8 percent. The most recent public health statistics show that so far in the 1970's, life expectancy has increased by 2.1 percent.

Numberless media messages have identified Amer-

ABOUT YOUR HEART AND YOUR HEALTH GENERALLY

ica's No. 1 killer as heart disease. Deaths due to cardiovascular failure reached a high point in the 1960's. Now, in the 1970's, the effectiveness of this killer has been reduced to the 1950's level.

The new commitment of millions of Americans to programs of increased physical fitness—especially aerobic exercise—has unquestionably played a major role in this dramatic turnaround.

Despite the improved statistics just noted, the airwaves remain crammed with messages about the dangers of heart disease as the No. 1 national killer. Heart disease *is* a national problem, and we should be concerned with everything we can do about it. But perhaps fewer scare words and a little more informal discussion of the problem would be helpful.

The words "heart disease" encompass many and varied conditions. Some are of real concern and others are of no significance at all. It is of the utmost importance that anyone carrying the label of "heart disease" know, if possible, the exact nature of the ailment and any limitations of activity that go along with it.

A few decades ago the diagnosis of heart disease was considered by many to be a sentence to a lifetime of semi-invalidism and early death. Fortunately, this concept no longer prevails. We know that heart disease is frequently compatible with living a normal, productive life with minimal, if any, restrictions. In fact, many people who have identifiable heart problems find that the adoption of more sensible living habits not only ameliorates their illness but also

CHAPTER 8

creates widespread benefits in all their spheres of activity.

Let me state again that there are many conditions that could loosely be called heart disease with which you could live to a very ripe old age.

I met one man with "heart disease" on a golf course. Play was slow that day, and we talked while we waited. He asked me what digitalis was for. He said he didn't know why he was taking this drug because he jogged two miles a day, was on the go all the time, worked hard, played a lot of golf, always walked and pulled a cart, and nothing in the way of exertion ever bothered him. That day he was playing 36 holes.

"They ran me on a treadmill," he said, "and said my heart was working fine as far as the coronary arteries were concerned, and still they put me on digitalis. I don't understand it."

I said I didn't know why that drug had been prescribed, but that I assumed he had some irregularity in his heartbeat, perhaps a certain kind of skipping, and that the easiest and best treatment for this is often digitalis.

What is tough for me to believe is that my friend's doctor did not explain fully what his condition was and what effect the medication would have on it. For whatever reason, what stuck in his mind was what he had heard or imagined about digitalis, instead of what his doctor had told him. Digitalis had become a scare word to him.

You probably have heard or read about the warning signs that the body sends when there is something wrong with the way your cardiovascular system is working. I want to repeat them. Of course, there are conditions that don't send out any signals at all, but if you become aware of any of the following symptoms, you should consult your doctor.

See your doctor if:

1. You are inordinately out of breath after having climbed one flight of stairs, or if you feel pain or tightness in your chest during any exertion or excitement. Discomfort in the chest may have nothing to do with your heart; extra pressure—gas in the stomach or intestine—may cause pain when the heart is completely well. But if you bet it's just gas or indigestion when it isn't, that would be a big bet to lose. So play it safe and see your doctor. Some warning signals are more serious than others. A burning in the chest, which may or may not be what is commonly called heartburn, is one of these, especially if it is felt in the neck and jaw, too. It may go away after you rest for a while, but it still warrants a trip to the doctor. If the pain is felt in the arms and shoulders, or the elbows, see him all the sooner.

2. Swelling of the feet and ankles suggests that your circulatory system may not be up to par (what most people are trying to get their golf game *down* to).

So does persistent and chronic fatigue. Just because you may be getting older doesn't mean you have to put up with being tired most of the time.

3. Evidence of impaired circulation may show up in the form of cramps in your legs when you are cycling

or jogging. Be sure to check this symptom with your doctor.

These are things that you have to know, but don't let them worry or upset you unduly. If it turns out that you have a condition that requires disciplined attention, you will join more than ten million other Americans who have similar problems and yet continue to lead very active and productive lives.

Dramatic advances have been made in the last decade in the research, diagnosis, treatment and control of heart disease. Progress has made it possible for thousands and thousands of people to survive and recover from heart and blood-vessel afflictions. Brilliant surgical practices for correcting certain heart defects have been developed, and we look for greater advances in the future.

As important as medical miracles is the fact that a damaged body has an almost unbelievable potential for curing itself—*if given a chance under proper direction.*

The history of golf has many inspiring examples of the ability of the human body to repair and restore itself, especially with the assistance of determination and discipline.

Amazing in his comeback was Ben Hogan, who was nearly destroyed in an automobile accident in 1949. He was given little chance of living and no hope of ever playing golf again. Hogan refused to accept that verdict and, by sheer will and courage, worked himself back to championship performance.

More recently, Gene Littler, in April, 1972, survived radical cancer surgery, at age forty-one. His condition demanded the removal of major muscles of the chest and back, as well as of the nerve supply to these areas. Immediately after the operation, Gene recalls that he couldn't move his left arm at all. After being discharged from the hospital, he went right to work on a rehabilitation program.

The weeks went by and, as one of his doctors said, "Gene is such a good athlete, his integration of muscle activity so automatic, so flexible, that he can lose a muscle or two and compensate enough to fool almost anybody." The physician went on to identify Littler as "one of the most conscientious, hardest working patients I've ever had."

Reserved and serious, Gene Littler is a quiet man who doesn't talk much, but who has always taken good care of himself. He credited much of his recovery to that and to swimming every day, in addition to the specially prescribed exercises.

In July, 1972, Gene accepted an invitation to the one-day pro-am Armstrong Cork Invitational. He birdied the last two holes and won the tournament. Since then, he has played in many tournaments, winning the St. Louis Classic in 1973 and the Japanese Masters in 1974, the year he was inducted into the World Golf Hall of Fame. But he was still waiting to pass the kind of grueling test he knew he would have to, if he were going to prove to himself that he was as good as ever.

That challenge came during the 1977 Bing Crosby

CHAPTER 8   National Pro-Am, played on three of the toughest courses in the world. Gene won it. He was back. Proudly, he said, "I figure I can win anywhere now."

Nothing is more important for you to believe in than the almost miraculous resources of your body to respond to a carefully designed conditioning program.

9: The Aerobic Exercises

IF YOU HAD TO PLACE emphasis on just one aspect of good conditioning, it might well be increasing your ability to deliver and better utilize oxygen in all parts of the body. That's what aerobic exercises are all about.

JOGGING/RUNNING

Much has been written about the difference between running and jogging. Some authorities maintain that you are jogging when you can carry on a conversation with someone jogging along with you. I suppose this suggests two things: one, that if you are jogging, you have enough breath left over to talk; and, two, that if

CHAPTER 9

your companion is running while you are jogging, pretty soon your companion will be beyond the sound of your voice.

From my point of view, this is a distinction without a difference. Both jogging and running involve man's oldest method of getting from one place to another. Automobile manufacturers have managed to make their product synonymous with "personal transportation." If you want *really* personal transportation, try your legs.

If you are just starting an exercise program, a good general rule is that the older you are the easier you should do *any* of the exercises. Your body knows its capacity better than you do. Pay attention to what it tells you.

Here is a perfectly good way to start. Get in your car and calculate distance on a local road of your choice. Use some roadside objects as markers at a half mile, mile and so on as far as you like.

Buy a good pair of shoes designed expressly for running—not just any shoes will do. Dr. George Sheehan says favorable things about the Puma 9190, Nike Cortez and Tiger, and the New Balance Trackster III. There are others, of course. What you want is a good-sized heel with a strong heel counter, a multilayered sole to handle shock, and a solid shank.

What you wear matters little. But if it's cold, several layers of light clothing are better than one bulky jacket.

Now that you are all equipped, go outdoors and start. Begin your measured course at a fast walk—

about 50 steps. Then jog 50. Then walk again and jog again, and so on. Take it easy and let the distance increase and the time you cover it in decrease gradually and naturally—but with a little improvement on every outing. Keep track of the distance you cover and the time you spent doing it. This is a race you are bound to win. You can only lose by not doing it at all. Of course, the idea is to demand more and more of your performance, and the prize is getting in shape to play the best golf of your life—and to feel better about life generally.

Jogging programs are particularly subject to dropouts. When you jog, your entire body weight pounds down on first one foot and then the other. Few people are conditioned to do much of this without a pre-training period of considerable duration. Many doctors have reported a very high incidence of shin splints, heel spurs, Achilles tendonitis and knee problems as a direct result of doing too much jogging too soon. The same sort of side effects may result from skipping rope and jumping-jack exercises, but bicycling produced the same aerobic results with none of these dangers. Whichever you choose, though, don't overdo it at first. Remember, this program is designed to improve your golf game and your health, not destroy them. Don't be eager for more good results than your body is capable of achieving. You'll feel a lot better sooner than you think possible, but don't rush into it at first.

Dr. Sheehan, who is known to all readers of *The Physician and Sports Medicine* magazine as a "running

CHAPTER 9

doctor," began running and writing about it twelve years ago. Although he maintains that running is the best exercise of all, he has some of the same reservations I have. He wrote, "Running shortens calf, hamstring and low back muscles. It also causes relative weakness of the abdominal muscles . . . daily exercises should give you permanent and pain-free running."

The major point this book is trying to make is that almost all the 600 or so muscles of your body are involved in your golf swing. Our goal is to tone them *evenly* and not to concentrate on the development of any single muscle area to the neglect of others.

SKIPPING ROPE

This exercise most of you will remember from seeing pictures of boxers in training. There are plenty of good reasons for doing it. It not only strengthens the heart and increases your endurance, it conditions leg and arm muscles as well as improving your posture and coordination. More than any other exercise we recommend, skipping rope increases your agility. When you add to these benefits the fact that your whole body is participating in an exercise that depends on a sense of rhythm and timing, it is obvious how beneficial it could be to your golf game.

The equipment is minimal. All you need is a length of rope about 8½ feet long. Adjust the length according to the illustration.

THE AEROBIC EXERCISES

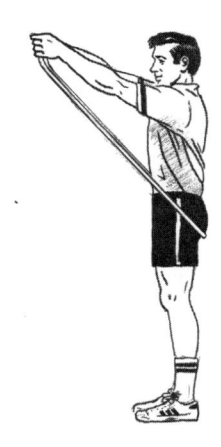

Hold the ends of the rope in your hands, loop it under your buttocks and stretch the rope as indicated. Knot the rope at the proper length.

Those of you who have never indulged in skipping rope or who haven't done so since your pre-teens may find this a very tough exercise when you first try it. The trick is to keep the rope in motion with the smallest possible circular movements of the wrist joints. As always, take it easy at the beginning and gradually increase the number of minutes you spend doing it.

BICYCLING

Combined with the basic isotonics, it is hard to fault bicycling as an all-around conditioning exercise. It conditions heart, lungs, legs and important musculature in the lower abdomen and back. By all means do as much bicycling as you can. However, if you don't know the bicycle safety rules of the road in your community, be sure to learn them before you begin.

Terrain and climate in many areas of the country may make outdoor bicycling impossible during several months of the year—a limitation it shares with golf. Consequently, as a year-around conditioning routine it is fortunate that the stationary bicycle, or exercycle, offers all the benefits of the outdoor road machine, with none of its handicaps. The stationary bike is available for use at any time and in any weather in any part of the country. It can be adjusted for difficulty of pedaling and many models have odometers to measure distance "traveled."

The common objection people have to bicycling in place is that it is boring. This is true only if you let it be true. Don't forget, your bike is portable. You can put it in any room of the house, on the deck or porch, on the patio, in your garden, next to the pool, facing an open door, or in your game room in front of the TV set. Some dedicated fans of stationary bike riding read while they cycle. Others listen to their radios or stereos. One can relax and enjoy without being concerned with traffic, turn signals, obstacles ahead, or any of the matters of road cycling.

Combining exercises is fun and productive if you have a stationary bike. For example, you can use the rubber grips on the handlebars to do your hand exercises. Another exercise you can do while pedaling is to contract and release the abdominal muscles. Imagination is the key to the enjoyment and rewards of this excellent conditioner.

THE AEROBIC EXERCISES

Start every session easily. Remember that your heart needs to be warmed up as well as your other muscles. Use the bicycle's drag adjustment to suit your developing capability, but don't start the next session at the same degree of difficulty—build up to it.

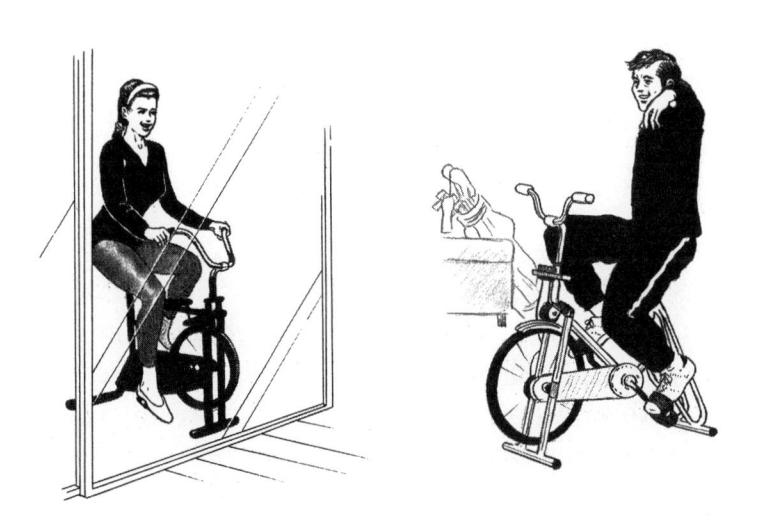

10: Aquadynamics

THIS IS THE WORD for doing exercises in the water. Again, climate and availability of places to swim control how much of this you can do. Since 1965, new in-ground pools have been built at the rate of about 80,000 per year. It is estimated that at present there are more than a million and a half swimming pools available across the country. The majority are residential, but about 400,000 are in colleges, schools, athletic clubs and public recreation facilities. In addition, there are more than two million above-ground pools.

Most of the recommended basic exercises can be performed in water that is waist deep, so don't underestimate the potential of a small, inexpensive backyard pool. Of course, if a lake or ocean is handy you have no problem at all, except when the water is too cold. In Vermont, unfortunately, this is most of the year.

Begin by doing your familiar warm-up set, then get in the water and be aquadynamic. Do the exercises in the order suggested. The first four you can do waist deep in the ocean or a lake without anything to hang on to. The last three require a pretty well filled pool of some kind.

Swimming in and of itself can be an almost perfect exercise, especially in that people with varying degrees of physical tolerance can use it to develop organic vitality and improve flexibility, strength and blood circulation.

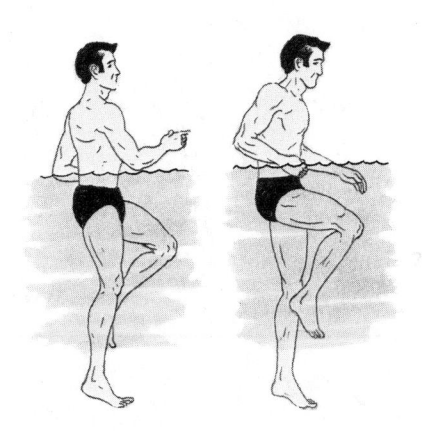

1. JOGGING IN PLACE

Standing with arms bent in running position, swimmer:
(1) Jogs in place.
    One minute.

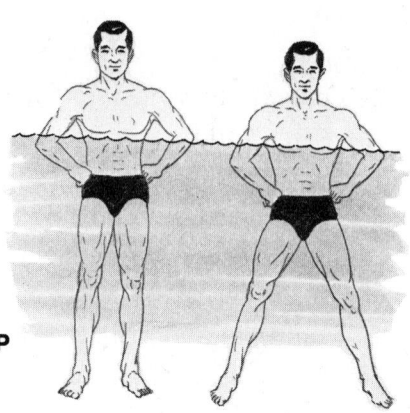

2. SIDE STRADDLE HOP

Standing in waist- to chest-deep water with hands on hips, swimmer:
(1) Jumps sideward to position with feet approximately 2 feet apart.
(2) Recovers.
  30 seconds.

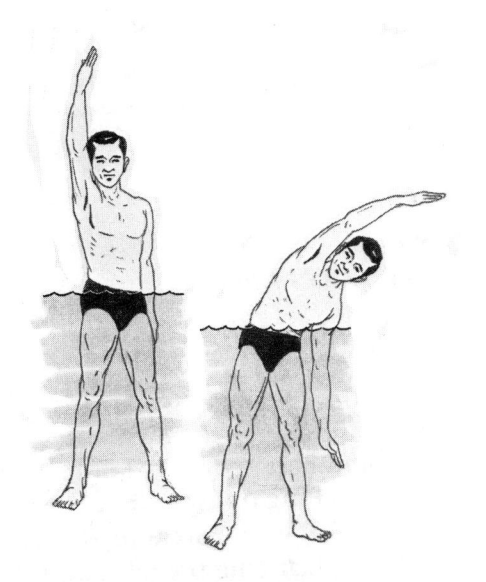

3. SIDE BENDER

Standing in waist-deep water with left arm at side and right arm overhead, swimmer:
(1) Stretches, slowly bending to the left.
(2) Recovers to the starting position.
Repeat.
Reverse to right arm at side and left arm overhead.
30 seconds.

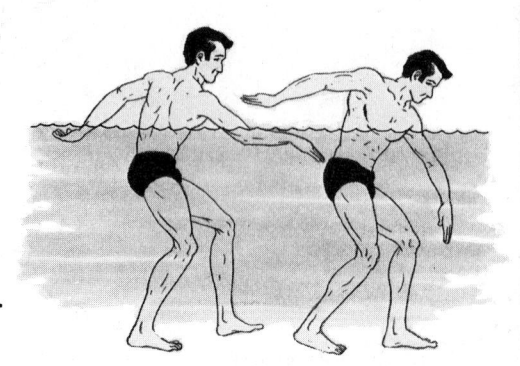

CHAPTER 10

4. STANDING CRAWL

Standing in waist- to chest-deep water, swimmer:

Simulates the overhand crawl stroke by:
(1) Reaching out with left hand, getting a grip on the water, pressing downward and pulling, bringing the left hand through to the thigh.
(2) Reaching out with the right hand, etc. Repeat.

30 seconds.

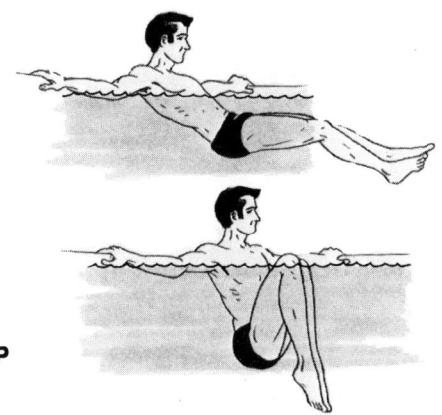

5. POOL-SIDE KNEES UP

Supine, holding onto pool gutter with hands and legs extended, swimmer:
(1) Brings knees to chin.
(2) Recovers to starting position.
   Repeat.
   30 seconds.

CHAPTER 10

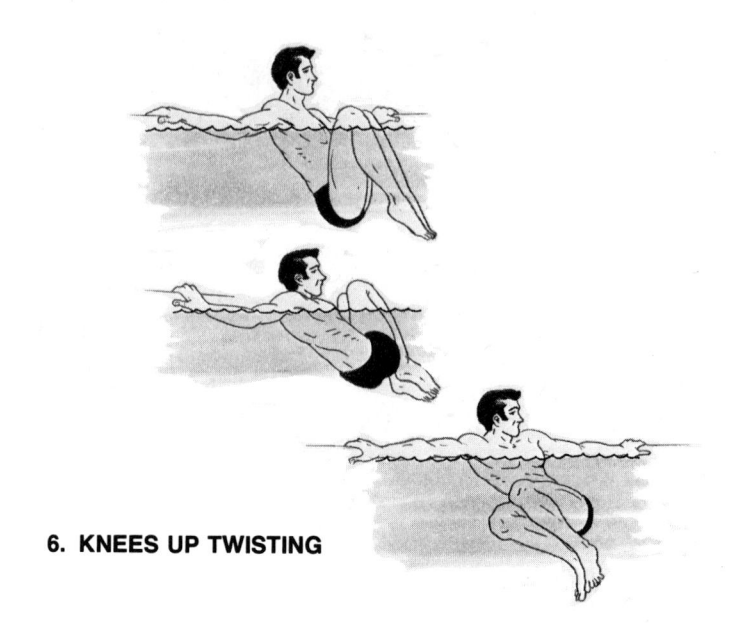

6. KNEES UP TWISTING

Supine, holding onto pool edge with knees drawn up to chest, swimmer:
(1) Twists slowly to left.
(2) Recovers.
(3) Twists slowly to right.
(4) Recovers.
   Repeat.
   30 seconds.

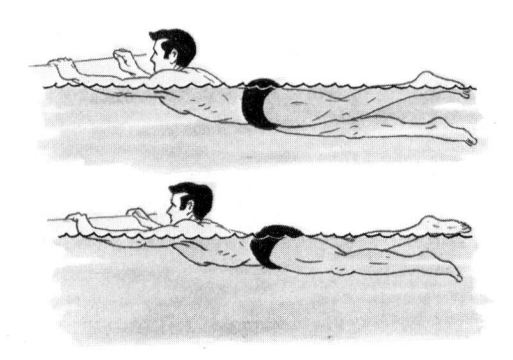

7. FRONT FLUTTER KICKING

Lying in a prone position and holding onto side of pool with hand(s), swimmer:
(1) Kicks flutter style so that toes are pointed back, ankles flexible, knee joints loose but straight, the whole leg acting as a whip. 30 seconds.

8. BACK FLUTTER KICKING

Turn over from front flutter kicking and repeat same movements.

This introductory set of water exercises, as described and timed, is, of course, isotonic rather than aerobic. It is you who make the exercises aerobic by the length of time and how vigorously you repeat them. Let your developing capacity be your guide, but increase the time as rapidly as possible. Also, swim

CHAPTER 10

as frequently and as long as you can. Just like your golf swing, swimming involves almost all the muscles of your body.

11: The Isometric Exercises

ISOMETRICS IS THE NEW WORD for what Charles Atlas promoted more than 50 years ago as the routine of "pitting muscle against muscle." The method has many values, especially for developing specific muscles or muscle groups. Try isometrics, if you like, except if you are on a limited exercise schedule designed by your doctor because of a known medical condition. If that is the case, follow his advice.

Isometric contraction exercises take very little time and require no special equipment. They're excellent muscle strengtheners and, as such, are valuable supplements to the rest of the program we've outlined.

The idea of isometrics is to work out a muscle by pushing or pulling against an immovable object such as a wall, or by pitting it against the opposition of another muscle.

The basis is the "overload" principle of exercise physiology, which holds that a muscle required to perform work beyond the usual intensity will grow in strength. Research indicates that one hard, 6- to 8-second isometric contraction per workout can, over a period of six months, produce a significant strength increase in a muscle.

The exercises illustrated and described in the following pages cover major large-muscle groups of the body. They can be performed almost anywhere and at almost any time. There is no set order for doing them, nor do all of them have to be completed at one time. You can, if you like, do one or two in the morning and others at various times during the day whenever you have half a minute or even less to spare.

For each contraction, maintain tension no more than eight seconds. Do little breathing during a contraction; breathe deeply between contractions.

Start easily. Do not apply maximum effort in the beginning. For the first three or four weeks, you should exert only about one-half of what you think is your maximum force. Use the first three or four seconds to build up to this degree of force, and the remaining four or five seconds to hold it.

For the next two weeks, gradually increase force until you reach nearly your maximum. After about six weeks, it will be safe to exert maximum effort.

Pain indicates you're applying too much force; reduce the amount immediately. If pain continues to accompany any exercise, discontinue using that exercise for a week or two. Then try it again with about 50 percent of maximum effort and, if no pain occurs, gradually build up toward maximum.

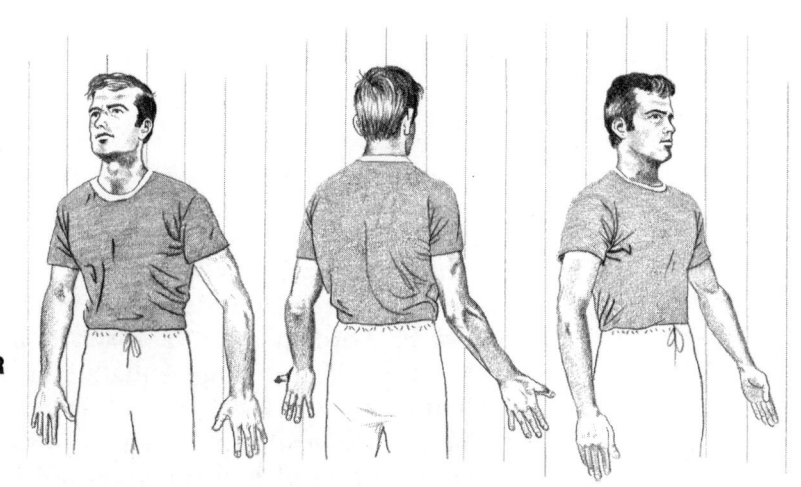

THE ISOMETRIC EXERCISES

UPPER BODY

1. *Starting position:* Stand, back to wall, hands at sides, palms toward wall.
   Action: Press hands backward against wall, keeping arms straight.
2. *Starting position:* Stand facing wall, hands at sides, palms toward wall.
   Action: Press hands forward against wall, keeping arms straight.
3. *Starting position:* Stand in doorway or with side against wall, arms at sides, palms toward legs.
   Action: Press hand(s) outward against wall or door frame, keeping palms straight.

CHAPTER 11

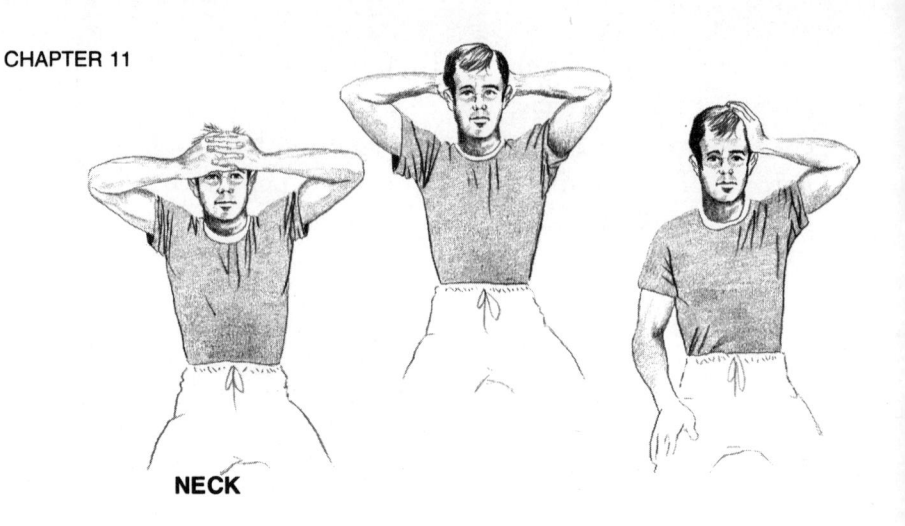

NECK

1. *Starting position:* Sit or stand, with interlaced fingers of hands on forehead.
   Action: Forcibly exert a forward push of head while resisting equally hard with hands.
2. *Starting position:* Sit or stand, with interlaced fingers of hands behind head.
   Action: Push head backward while exerting a forward pull with hands.
3. *Starting position:* Sit or stand, with palm of left hand on left side of head.
   Action: Push with left hand while resisting with head and neck. Reverse, using right hand on right side of head.

THE ISOMETRIC
EXERCISES

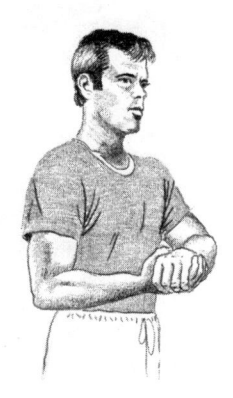

ARMS

Starting position: Stand with feet slightly apart. Flex right elbow, close to body, palm up. Place left hand over right.
Action: Forcibly attempt to curl right arm upward, while giving equally strong resistance with the left hand. Repeat with left arm.

CHAPTER 11

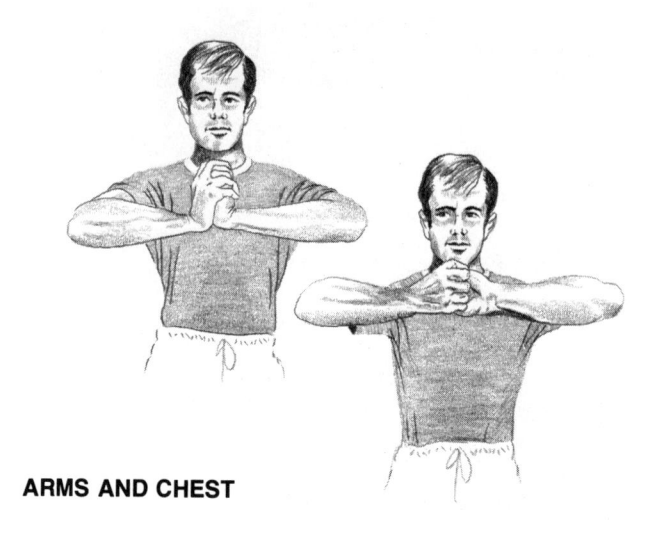

ARMS AND CHEST

1. *Starting position:* Stand with feet comfortably spaced, knees slightly bent. Clasp hands, palms together, close to chest.
   Action: Press hands together and hold.
2. *Starting position:* Stand with feet slightly apart, knees slightly bent. Grip fingers, arms close to chest.
   Action: Pull hard and hold.

As you do any of these exercises, keep in mind how important the *left side* is to your golf game. Most golfers are right-handed, which means that the hand, arm, shoulder and back muscles of the right side are more developed and are in better condition than corresponding muscles on the left side. In many cases, the right hand and forearm may be slightly larger than the left.

Concentrate particularly on the third of the upper body isometrics, which is great for the development of the extensor muscles of the arms. You can, to advantage, do the exercise for the left arm only whenever and wherever you care to. The idea, of course, is to equalize the muscle tone and strength of your left and right sides. Your right arm is accustomed to being dominant, but if you let it control the golf swing you'll get into trouble.

THE ISOMETRIC EXERCISES

12: Some Specific Golfing Exercises

WHICHEVER OF THE PREVIOUS exercise programs you choose to do, and how you choose to perform them, is entirely up to you. But, please, try to combine the indoor exercises with at least one kind of outdoor routine. It's our feeling that combining the isotonics with at least one of the aerobics will produce the quickest and best results in terms of both your golf and your overall health. Specific golf exercises alone will improve your shotmaking, but, combined with a full program of general physical conditioning, they will raise your performance to a level you probably never thought was possible.

You may have noticed that some players on the pro tour seem to swing so slowly that you wonder where the power is coming from. It is derived from club-

SOME SPECIFIC GOLFING EXERCISES

head speed, squarely applied, and it is primarily generated by hand and wrist action. There are several terms for this, the most common of which is "uncocking the wrists." Properly executed, the action takes place about halfway through the downswing. But most golfers do it from the *top* of the backswing, which robs them of both accuracy and distance.

To overcome that tendency, we suggest that you practice your swing with a weighted wood, possibly your driver or a three wood. You don't have to have the club altered in any way. There are now available, at your pro shop or via mail order, at least two pieces of special equipment designed for this purpose. One is a weighted club-head cover and the other is a lead "doughnut" device that slides down over the shaft. There are also special exercise clubs that your golf professional will be glad to tell you about.

Swing the weighted wood for a while and you'll feel the muscles that are directly involved in the uncocking of the wrists. Keep swinging whenever you can and you'll soon see the benefits in extra length and accuracy in all your shots.

There is a wonderful indoor exercise that you can do to supplement practice swinging. (When you first start doing this exercise, use one of your woods without any additional weight. You can always add weight when your muscles are ready for it.) Take your regular driving stance and hold the club exactly as if you were going to play the shot. Raise your arms to shoulder height, as in Figure 1.

CHAPTER 12

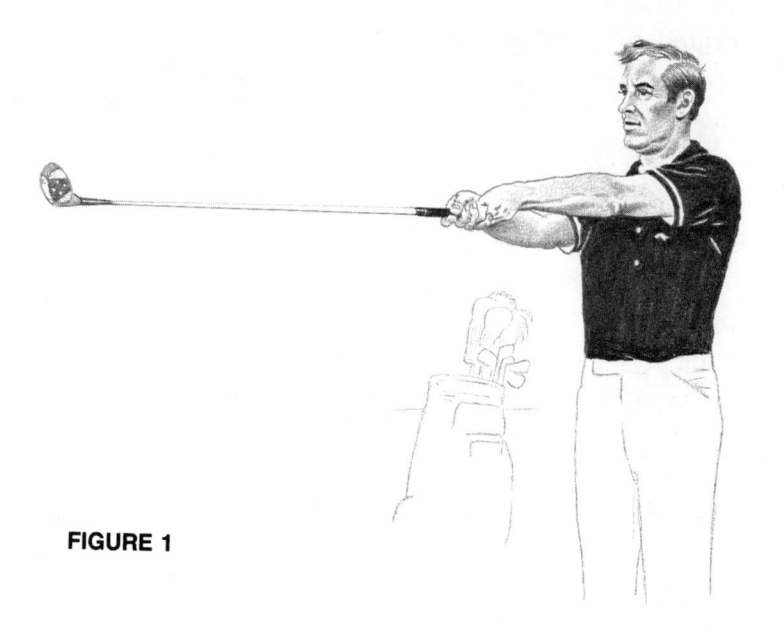

FIGURE 1

Now, keeping your arms stretched out, and without moving your body, cock your wrists as in Figure 2. Make sure that the club head stays in line with your shoulders and straight left arm. Hold the position briefly and return to the starting position. Don't worry about uncocking after you have struck the ball—the momentum of the swing will take care of that. Do the exercise in this position until it is almost automatic.

SOME SPECIFIC GOLFING EXERCISES

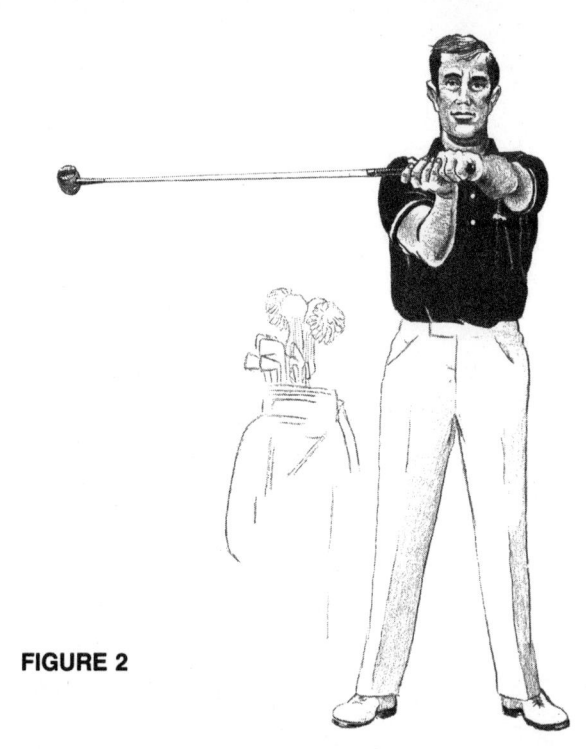

FIGURE 2

Then drop your arms to lower positions and repeat. Remember that the movement of the club *must* be kept in line with your straight left arm.

As we stressed earlier in the book, an exercise like this must be done correctly and with concentration, because we are not only trying to develop specific muscular capability, but also muscular *memory*. To realize the full potential of the specific golf exercises, they must be done repeatedly and precisely.

The exercise just described will make you conscious of the relative weakness of the third and fourth fingers of your left hand. Unless those fingers are equal partners in your grip with your right hand, your game will always be less powerful and more erratic than you'd like. Particularly if control of the club at the top of the swing is lost by those two fingers will you see much more of the woods and the water than any of your playing companions.

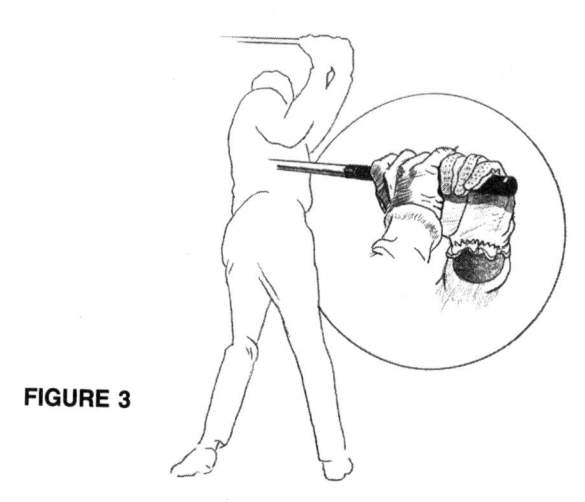

FIGURE 3

This exercise can be supplemented by a slightly different version that can be done sitting in a chair. With both arms bent and elbows held close to your sides, simply take your standard grip and lift the club up and down, moving nothing but your wrists in the cocking and uncocking motion. You might keep a spare club in your game room or study to tempt you to repeat this exercise during any odd moment of the day or evening.

Squeezing a rubber ball in each hand is an especially good exercise for the fingers and hands. You can use tennis balls for this routine, but they are not

SOME SPECIFIC GOLFING EXERCISES

as effective as plain rubber balls of a size that fits snugly in your hand. Work more with your left hand than your right to equalize their strength. Start by squeezing the balls rhythmically, using all fingers together. After a while, experiment with using the fingers one at a time in sequence. Ben Hogan believed in the ball-squeezing exercise, although he never performed it on a day he was going to compete.

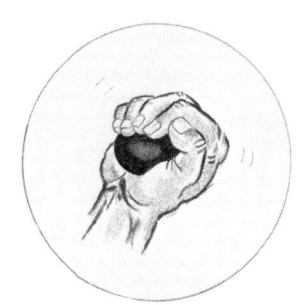

FIGURE 4

One great advantage of this hand exercise is that the balls can be carried with you and used when you are walking, jogging or riding the stationary bike.

I have a friend who likes to watch television but is infuriated by most of the commercial messages. He keeps a set of exercise balls handy and squeezes them to relieve his antagonism. He says it is good for his hands, his blood pressure and his sanity—and it also keeps him away from the refrigerator.

Speaking of blood pressure, we know that tension plays a major role in aggravating it. There are causes other than tension, but whatever the reason, proper exercise programs have proven over and over to be effective methods for lowering blood pressure.

13: Your Weight and What to Do About It

EVERY LABORATORY TECHNICIAN knows that lean rats live longer than fat rats. Furthermore, if the lean rats played golf, they'd probably play better golf, too. Carrying around excess weight robs you of vitality, puts an extra strain on your cardiovascular system, and does little for your appearance or your self-image. Weight control is a medical problem for some people, but for most of us it's a matter of choice.

You may already know all you care to about weight control. If not, I'd like to tell you that, like the attainment of so many worthwhile things in life, it is primarily a matter of desire and discipline. Maybe you are one of the thousands who try several different diets every year, lose a few pounds, prove to yourself that you can do it any time you feel like it—then

YOUR WEIGHT AND WHAT TO DO ABOUT IT

forget about the whole thing and gain all the weight back again.

You gain weight because your body stores up as fat the food it doesn't need. The more active you are, the less fat your body stores up. Predatory animals eat as much as they can hold whenever they have the opportunity. Their survival experience tells them they don't know when, or if, they are going to eat again. But they do know they will expend a lot of energy stalking their next prey.

In the zoological scheme of things, human beings are called *Homo sapiens,* which means wise or knowing man. In the affluent societies of the Western world, we are wise and knowing about a lot of things, but many of us apply little wisdom to our eating habits.

It is less than intelligent for people who want to lead active lives to eat so much at any one meal that all their available energy for a couple of hours is used up just digesting food. When the body recovers, it is faced with the choice of using the new energy or storing it.

It is just as simple as it sounds. All you have to do is adjust your energy intake to your energy outgo.

We are not going to talk about dieting. We are going to discuss the amount and kind of food you eat and how you spend the energy it creates. Money in the bank is one thing. Fat in the body bank is something else.

To give you an idea about what are considered to be desirable weights, look at the estimates in the accompanying tables.

CHAPTER 13

MEN OF AGES 25 AND OVER
Weight in Pounds According to Frame
(In Indoor Clothing)

HEIGHT (with shoes on) 1-inch heels Feet Inches		SMALL FRAME	MEDIUM FRAME	LARGE FRAME
5	2	112–120	118–129	126–141
5	3	115–123	121–133	129–144
5	4	118–126	124–136	132–148
5	5	121–129	127–139	135–152
5	6	124–133	130–143	138–156
5	7	128–137	134–147	142–161
5	8	132–141	138–152	147–166
5	9	136–145	142–156	151–170
5	10	140–150	146–160	155–174
5	11	144–154	150–165	159–179
6	0	148–158	154–170	164–184
6	1	152–162	158–175	168–189
6	2	156–167	162–180	173–194
6	3	160–171	167–185	178–199
6	4	164–175	172–190	182–204

If you are interested in losing weight, we have a great exercise for you. It's called *push away*. Push away from the table, the refrigerator, the bar, the popcorn machine, the snack bowls, the pastry cart, the hors d'oeuvres and the cookie jar. You might also remember the words of baseball's immortal Satchel Paige: "Don't eat fried foods, they just angry up the blood."

Stick to eating, every day, in *each* of the following groups.

DAIRY: whole, skim, evaporated or instant non-fat dry milk, buttermilk, cheese, ice cream, yogurt.

MEAT: meat, poultry, fish, eggs, dry beans, peas, nuts.

VEGETABLES/FRUITS: vitamin C-rich fruits or vegetables and at least one dark, leafy green, or yellow vegetable. Potatoes, too.

BREAD/CEREAL: whole grain or enriched cereals, noodles, rice and good bread, i.e., with nutritive value, as in whole wheat.

WOMEN OF AGES 25 AND OVER
Weight in Pounds According to Frame
(In Indoor Clothing)

HEIGHT (with shoes on) 2-inch heels Feet Inches		SMALL FRAME	MEDIUM FRAME	LARGE FRAME
4	10	92– 98	96–107	104–119
4	11	94–101	98–110	106–122
5	0	96–104	101–113	109–125
5	1	99–107	104–116	112–128
5	2	102–110	107–119	115–131
5	3	105–113	110–122	118–134
5	4	108–116	113–126	121–138
5	5	111–119	116–130	125–142
5	6	114–123	120–135	129–146
5	7	118–127	124–139	133–150
5	8	122–131	128–143	137–154
5	9	126–135	132–147	141–158
5	10	130–140	136–151	145–163
5	11	134–144	140–155	149–168
6	0	138–148	144–159	153–173

For girls between 18 and 25, subtract 1 pound for each year under 25.
Courtesy Metropolitan Life.

CHAPTER 13

Use as little processed sugar as possible. Fresh fruits, orange juice, raisins, dates and honey will help keep your blood sugar level where it should be. A candy bar or a drink of whiskey may give you a quick lift, but neither will stay with you long. If you are tempted by any, or all, of the hundreds of varieties of packaged junk foods, resist that temptation—they are almost completely composed of useless calories. Stay away, too, from those delicious morsels of fat on your meat. Why eat fat when that's what you are trying to get rid of?

If you really want to work out a weight-reducing program, you may be interested in the following estimates of caloric consumption keyed to various activities.

Note that the table is adjusted to a 150-pound person. Naturally, the more excess weight you are maintaining, the more energy you consume. Remember, all you have to do every week, unlike your bank account, is to take out more than you put in.

A calorie-count index can be found on page 111.

ENERGY EXPENDITURE BY A 150-POUND PERSON IN VARIOUS ACTIVITIES

Activity	Gross energy cost, Cal. per hr.
A. Rest and light activity	50–200
Lying down or sleeping	80
Sitting	100
Driving an automobile	120
Standing	140
Domestic work	180

Energy Expenditure by a 150-pound Person *(cont.)*

Activity	Gross energy cost, Cal. per hr.
B. Moderate activity	200–350
Bicycling (5½ mph)	210
Walking (2½ mph)	210
Gardening	220
Canoeing (2½ mph)	230
Golf	250
Lawn mowing (power mower)	250
Lawn mowing (hand mower)	270
Bowling	270
Fencing	300
Rowing (2½ mph)	300
Swimming (¼ mph)	300
Walking (3¾ mph)	300
Badminton	350
Horseback riding (trotting)	350
Square dancing	350
Volleyball	350
Roller skating	350
C. Vigorous activity	over 350
Table tennis	360
Ditch digging (hand shovel)	400
Ice skating (10 mph)	400
Wood chopping or sawing	400
Tennis	420
Water skiing	480
Hill climbing (100 ft. per hr.)	490
Skiing (10 mph)	600
Squash and handball	600
Cycling (13 mph)	660
Scull rowing (race)	840
Running (10 mph)	900

For the purpose of illustration, let's examine the calorie flow of an "average" person. During a 24-hour period, the number of calories expended might look something like this:

		Calories expended
Sleeping	8 hours	640
Driving car	2 hours	240
Sitting at work	6 hours	600
Standing	2 hours	280
Walking	1 hour	210
Working around house or yard	3 hours	540
Watching TV	2 hours	200
		2,710

Now, what did our "average" person eat during this period?

	Calories consumed
Breakfast: orange juice, two eggs, two slices buttered toast, coffee	550
Mid-morning snack: glass of milk, sweet roll or doughnut, coffee	400
Light lunch: cup of soup, tunafish sandwich, cola drink	600
Afternoon snack: candy bar and cola	500
Cocktail hour: a few potato chips, nuts and two cocktails	750
Simple dinner: apple juice, bread and butter, two hamburgers, mashed potatoes, lima beans and one slice of lemon meringue pie	1,525
Evening snack: popcorn and two beers	1,000
	5,325

YOUR WEIGHT AND WHAT TO DO ABOUT IT

Obviously, our "average" player lost this match by a wide margin, since about 2,600 calories were never used up. But when you do a little figuring, it begins to look as if the scoring system wasn't much good. For example, one pound generally translates into 3,500 calories. So theoretically, if one took in 2,500 more calories a day than one put out, at the end of a year 260 pounds would have been gained. It doesn't happen this way, of course, because different people expend energy in different ways and at different rates and digestion is rarely 100% efficient. Then there are the enviable ones who apparently can eat anything and as much as they want—and never put on a pound.

But suppose you are not one of the lucky ones and you have put on excess weight, what do you do about it? Again, the answer is simple: exercise more and eat less. This doesn't mean you have to pass up all the foods you like best. You can eat, drink and be merry and still bring your weight down by simply substituting fewer and better meals and giving up some of the goodies and in-between munchies.

Naturally, it will require time—and will power. You didn't gain the weight in ten days, and you must not try to melt it away in ten days.

Theoretically, if you have been eating at the rate of 5,000 calories a day and eat nothing at all for 10 days, you would lose 14 pounds. We can't promise that this will happen—and even if it did you wouldn't be in much shape to play golf at the end of the experiment. The truth is that some delicious foods have far fewer

CHAPTER 13

calories than others. We have included a calorie table in this book so that you can see for yourself what they are, and design your own eating program.

To show you how easy it is, let's go back to our friend, the "average" person. He could eat the same breakfast, but should eliminate the mid-morning sweet roll and substitute for it a large glass of orange juice. The natural sugar gives our friend the desired lift, in energy and spirit. Lunch is the same but the afternoon snack is skipped due to the approaching cocktail hour. This is enjoyed in the customary way, except that some nutritious cheese and crackers are exchanged for the potato chips and nuts.

The "simple" dinner menu changes. A baked potato is substituted for the mashed potato, broiled fish or chicken for the hamburgers and peas for the lima beans. Instead of luscious pie for dessert, an equally luscious melon or fresh-fruit compote is served.

During the evening's television session, our friend still has a couple of beers but instead of reaching for the popcorn bowl, the hands now keep busy with the exercise balls or the golf club that just happens to be propped by the TV set.

With a little effort and restraint, our player has cut about 2,500 calories from the day's total. The match is now just about even and, with a little more exercise, our friend can win. Undoubtedly, it takes some planning and definitely some self-control. But so does a good round of golf. Dining out at a neighbor's home is more difficult because you have no menu to order from, but if your hostess seems concerned that you didn't like the dinner she slaved over, you can always speak to her privately and explain.

If you explore the calorie table at the back of the book, you can find very quickly a wide variety of foods that you really enjoy. This will make all the difference in your weight-control program, because you'll find yourself looking forward to all the delicious foods you *can* eat, rather than being discouraged by the thought of what you *shouldn't* eat. In a way, it's like your golf swing: the sooner a habit pathway is formed, the sooner you can forget about the details.

You can speed up your fitness program by taking advantage of every opportunity to supplement it during the course of the day. If you have a lawn and garden to maintain, think about staying away from laborsaving devices, like self-propelled lawn mowers and you-don't-have-to-bend-over clipping equipment. Do as much as you can with your own power. You'll improve muscle tone and capability and use up calories at the same time.

Here are other specific suggestions:

—Stairs versus elevator or escalator. At least now and then, choose the stairs. Take two at a time as often as possible.

—Breaks. Along with, or instead of, those mid-morning or mid-afternoon time-outs for coffee, take exercise breaks. No need to get into a sweat. Do a

CHAPTER 13

conditioning exercise or two, if convenient. If you lack privacy, do some of the inconspicuous isometric exercises.

—Pull-ins. Suck in your abdomen now and then and hold it taut for a few seconds.

—Up for a stretch. If you must work in a static, sitting position, get up occasionally, stand erect, stretch a bit and move around.

—Rub away. After a shower or bath, towel yourself vigorously. That's exercise, too, stimulating for muscles as well as skin.

14: Some Pointers to Playing Better

As a doctor and an avid student of the game of golf, I do have some definite comments and suggestions which may be helpful in improving your game and the enjoyment you take in it.

Let's begin by taking a good, long look at the finished product in its ideal form.

Study these drawings of a fine, full, golf swing. Don't think about the anatomy or the mechanics involved. The last thing you should have in your mind, after you have played a bad shot, is whether or not it was caused by a malfunction of one of the *Latissimus dorsi* or a failure to properly advance the *Osinominatum*.

CHAPTER 14

USE YOUR POWERS OF VISUALIZATION

Look at the drawings of this swing long enough, and often enough, to imprint them on your mind. Then visualize yourself doing what you see. The human brain is the finest, most complex computer imaginable. Somehow, a visual input like this can be translated into neuromuscular response without conscious direction. You will never be able to program your system to figure out, consciously, how to hit a ball exactly 156 yards, or how firmly to strike a putt that has to travel 14 feet 6 inches and break 13½ inches to drop into the cup. Success in shotmaking is first and foremost a combination of sensory perception (especially visual) and muscle memory.

Think for a moment of the first few times you played catch with a child. Perhaps you were 10 feet apart. How did the child learn just how hard to toss the ball so it would reach your outstretched hands? The answer is simple. He kept on trying until he succeeded. His eyes observed and his whole muscular and nervous system reacted. When you increased the distance, the child didn't have to rethink the whole operation, he began to compensate *automatically.*

Golf can be learned in exactly the same way. Coordination is the combination of a number of muscles into a smooth pattern. The development of coordination depends on the repetition of this precisely performed pattern. As the activity is visualized and repeated many times, a habit pathway is formed and the activity can be performed with less and less conscious awareness of the particular elements that go to make the whole. During motor activities the brain is aware of the *general* performance of the body rather than the precise function of each muscle, tendon and joint.

Many golfers who, for whatever reason, may not have played the game for a long time have been pleasantly surprised by how well they performed the first time out. Figuratively, they had pressed the button marked GOLF SWING and it worked fine. After a while, though, they played a few bad shots and tried to make conscious corrections in the mechanics of their swings. The harder they tried and the more corrections they made, the more bad shots they hit. What they did was to interrupt their own miraculous muscle memory. Familiar habit pathways were blocked by conflicting conscious instructions until their whole game went to pieces.

Of course you'll have to practice what you visualize. Over and over. Either at a practice range or in your backyard or both. The exercises in this book will help greatly in doing that effectively. The better shape the muscles, tendons, ligaments and joints are in, the sooner they will coordinate in a habit pathway.

HOLDING THE CLUB

A good swing is illustrated on the next two pages. Look at it again. Now study these illustrations of a fine golf grip. We include them because no single factor in golf is as important as the way you hold the club. Do it correctly and there is no limit to how well you can play with practice and perseverance. Grip incorrectly and you will never pass beyond the duffer stage.

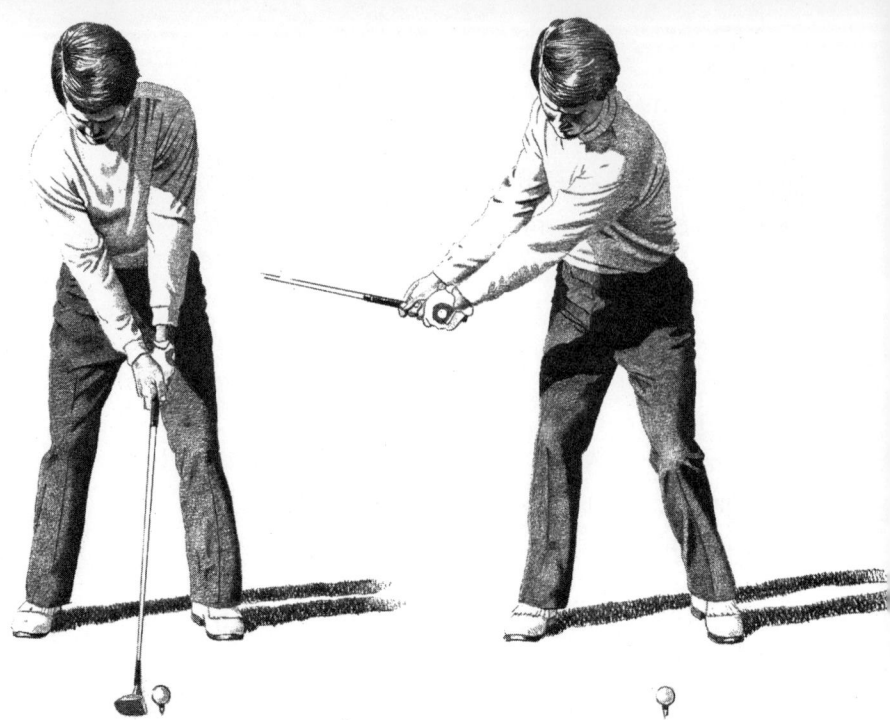

We have made a detailed study of the overlapping grip because it is used by the majority of golfers, both amateur and professional.

The interlocking grip is different, basically, only in one respect: the fourth finger of the right hand, instead of overlapping the first finger of the left hand, interlocks with it.

I should perhaps point out that no two grips are exactly alike any more than any two swings are. The

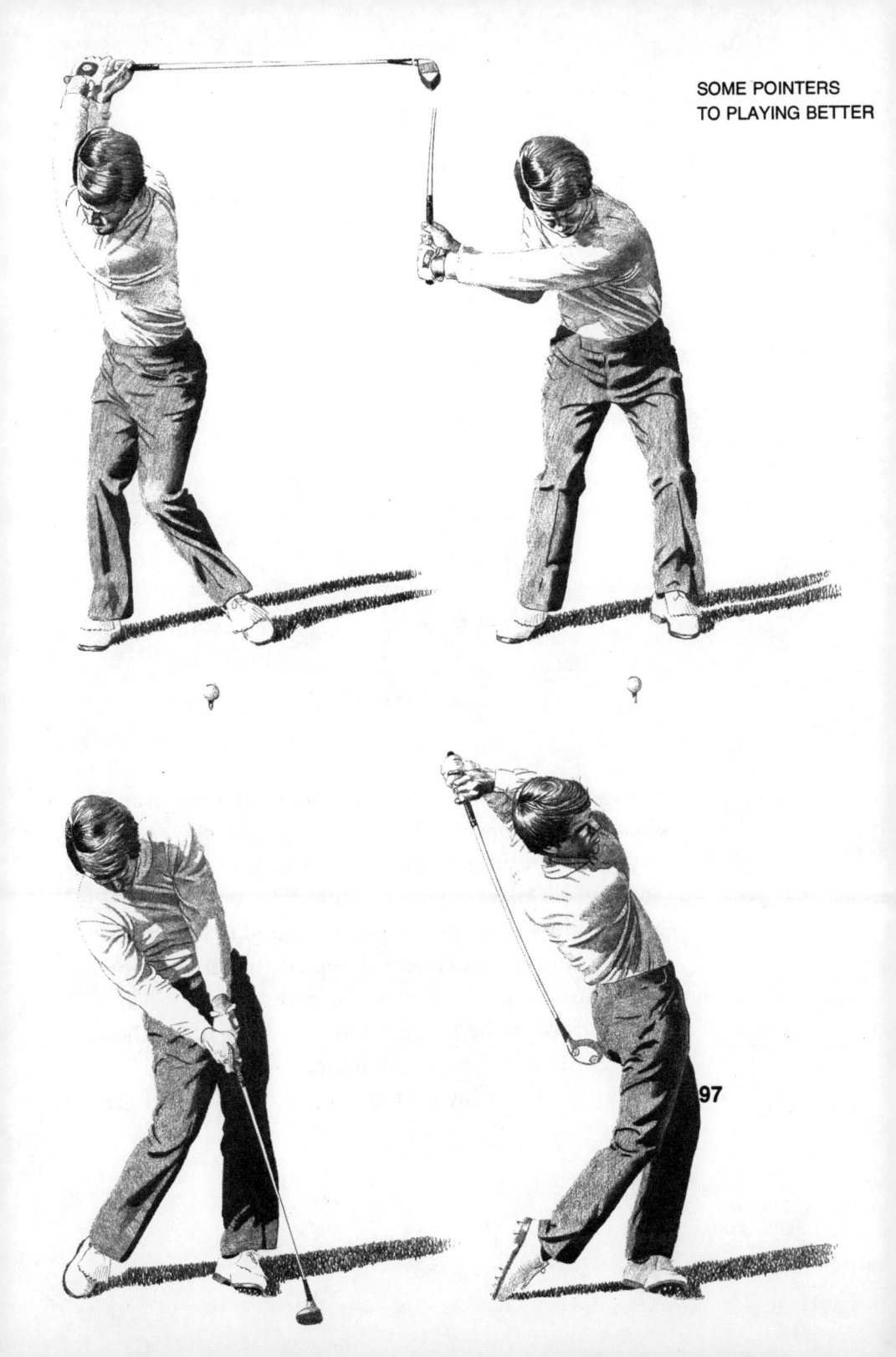

SOME POINTERS TO PLAYING BETTER

CHAPTER 14

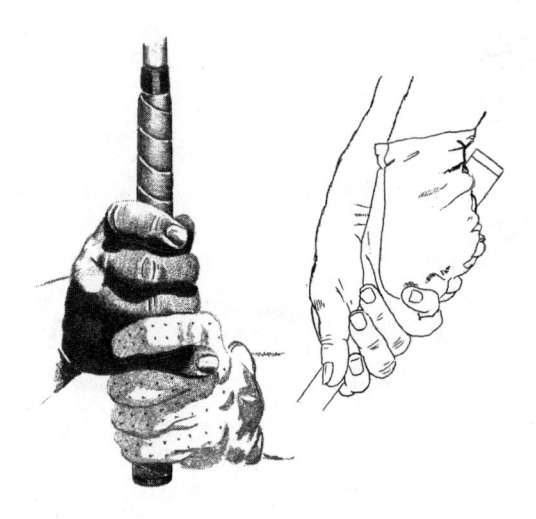

size of your hands and the length of your fingers dictate variations on the model we have shown—for instance, the interlocking grip has been chosen by some great players with small hands. Whatever grip you choose should *generally* correspond to the grip we have examined so closely. I repeat that if you don't learn how to grip the club correctly and *stick with it,* you'll probably be taking lessons all your life without having them do you much good.

You will probably find at first that the correct grip

feels uncomfortable and ineffective. Your hands will feel better in something approaching the baseball grip. In the long history of golf there have been a few players who were successful with the unlapped grip. *Your* chances of being successful with it are about as good as your chances of winning the Irish Sweepstakes. So you should concentrate on either an overlapping or an interlocking grip until your muscles almost refuse to hold the club any other way. And they will—just trust them.

Now visualize the swing again—*without* looking back at the illustration. Your professional will have explained the separate parts of it. No two good golf swings are identical, any more than any two human bodies are identical. Your body, once it knows exactly what is required of it, will design your own best swing.

One last comment on the grip. Many players grip the shaft of the club as if they were trying to strangle it. Try to keep in mind the notion that there is something inside the handle of the club that you'll crush if you squeeze it too hard. Too tight a grip will decrease both distance and accuracy. In a previous chapter, exercises were recommended to strengthen the muscles and tendons of the hands and forearms. You may now be wondering why you should do these if you are supposed to grip the club lightly. The answer is simple. It takes strong fingers and hands with well-developed sensitivity to be both firm *and* gentle. Weak hands are the ones most likely to squeeze too hard. Too tight a grip will make the proper hand and wrist action physically impossible.

CHAPTER 14

AIMING

Lining up the shot is one of the most important techniques in golf. The ball doesn't go where you wish or hope it will go, but only where you hit it. To be sure that you aim it correctly your mind needs the most precise information it can get from your two eyes working together.

Don't study a shot from an angle to your intended target line. Approach the ball directly from behind, facing the exact line you want it to travel. Hold this line with your eyes and place your club behind the ball so that the face of the club is at a right angle to the line you have chosen. Then take your stance, *without moving the club head.* In other words, adjust your stance to the position of the club head, not vice versa, as many players unfortunately do.

Many golfers, while going through this sequence, follow the target line back to a particular spot—a tuft of grass, a leaf—a few feet ahead of the ball on the same line. They concentrate on making certain that the ball passes over this spot after it leaves the club head.

This alignment technique is of supreme importance in putting. Pick a spot that the ball *must* go over if it is to hit the hole. Then putt for the spot. Sensory input and the muscle memory of thousands of putts will take care of the force factor.

SOME POINTERS TO PLAYING BETTER

YOU DON'T NEED FORCE TO HIT A GOLF BALL

Sometimes I feel that it is unfortunate that what you hit a golf ball with is usually called a club. The use of the word *stick* might avoid some damaging unconscious connotations. The effect of early conditioning in the use of a club is frequently apparent on practice ranges and fairways, where golfers seem to be trying to beat the ball to death before it gets away. One of the first things to get into your head when you begin to play golf is that you don't have to hurry or force your swing. The golf ball is going to stay right there waiting for the arrival of the club head, and the thing that will send it away is smooth club-head motion, not strength.

This might suggest that, because the ball is stationary when you hit it, golf should be an easier game to learn than, say, baseball or tennis, because you don't have to make instant adjustments to compensate for a curve or a bad bounce. Actually, it doesn't seem to work that way. The golfer with his motionless ball has more time for tension to build and for his mind to confuse the muscles with instructions.

TAKE A LESSON NOW AND THEN

If you are now playing golf regularly but haven't seen your teaching professional for a year or so, take a lesson. Amateurs, club pros—even touring pros—occasionally need help from an objective, knowledgeable observer. The best of them—Nicklaus, Palmer, Watson and others—have gratefully reported how another pro spotted something in their swing or grip that needed adjustment. This is fundamental to serious play. As the saying goes, "If you want a white fence, you have to paint it every so often."

SWINGING RHYTHMICALLY

Some people seem to have a better sense of rhythm than others, but even if you don't think you have a natural sense of rhythm, cheer up, you can acquire it.

Many fine golfers, Gene Sarazen included, firmly believe that the rhythm of the golf swing is the waltz rhythm: *one,* two, three, *one,* two, three, *one,* two, three, and so on. It works for a lot of good golfers. Try it, because it may work well for you.

Take your driving stance and start thinking waltz. Pick a tune you know well. Many golfers like "Take Me Out to the Ball Game." It works like this. Start your backswing with the word "Take." Swing slowly so the "Me" beat is at the top of your swing. The third count, the "Out," comes halfway through the downswing when your wrists start to uncock and begin to whip the club head through the ball—not *at* it, *through* it. Keep right on with the song and keep swinging. If you don't know all the words, make some up. One man we know has written a full set of words to the song beginning with "Take Me Out to the Golf Course."

The first result that you will notice from waltzing your swing is that you'll stop hitting from the top, an error that plagues most weekend golfers.

Some golfers like to practice the waltz swing to the tune of "The Merry Widow." That particular melody works like this: da, de, DA, de, da, de, DA, de, da, da, da. The DA in this tune corresponds to the "Out."

One good way to make this rhythm a natural part of your golf swing is to perform the body and shoulder-turn exercise to the same rhythm. After a while, the rhythm will become the natural way you hit a golf shot and make a great difference in how well you play.

PRACTICING

Someone once used the word "lucky" in congratulating Gary Player on a championship win. "Well, you know," said Gary, "it's a funny thing. The more I practice, the luckier I get."

Nobody—but nobody—has ever played this game well without a considerable amount of practice.

Swinging a club with the proper grip, especially the weighted one, is good for starters, but nothing replaces the actual experience of feeling the club head strike the ball and seeing the results.

If you care to buy a net and a driving mat, you can set up your own practice range in your cellar or your

CHAPTER 14

yard. This is far better than not practicing at all, but going to an outdoor range is much more productive.

There are all kinds of driving ranges, some good, some not so good. See if you can find one within easy driving distance of your home so you can get there on short notice when you have the impulse and the time.

Of course, you will take your own clubs with you. The first thing to look for is a level grassy area from which you can play iron shots and fairway woods. If there isn't one, you'll have to start from one of the tees, which may or may not provide a mat. If you are stuck with a range that has neither an area of turf nor a mat, you'd be well advised to work only with your woods and your long irons. Let's assume your practice facility, public or at your club, has an area where there is something resembling a piece of fairway from which to shoot.

Start by doing a few body bends and twists, then swing a couple of clubs to warm up your wrists and hands. Next, hit slow and easy practice shots, starting with your wedge. How many shots you hit, through the range of your irons, depends on how much time you have. One thing you can't learn too much about on public practice ranges is distance. The practice balls are mostly old, tired and lopsided. So don't worry much about the 250-yard marker—with those balls, even Jack Nicklaus couldn't reach it. Concentrate instead on your accuracy. That's where practice pays off the quickest.

If you don't hit each practice shot with as much care and concentration as you do on the course, don't

SOME POINTERS TO PLAYING BETTER

bother to practice at all. You'd be better off watching television and doing the wrist or hand exercises. Pick a spot where you want the ball to drop, line up your shot, visualize the flight line and make your swing. Then put another ball down and do it again. Remember that the longer the shot, the less accurate you will be as far as distance is concerned, so try to make up for this handicap by hitting the ball exactly on the line you have chosen.

If you are shooting for, say, the 175-yard marker, the matter of club selection becomes important. Forgetting, for the moment, the matter of the condition of the balls you are practicing with, listen to the advice of one of the greatest golfers of all time, Harry Vardon. He always advised the selection of a club *you know you can get there with*. Don't be influenced by the fact that the young lions are hitting the green on 200-yard, par-3 holes with five irons. That's probably beyond your capabilities. Remember that no one can beat you just by being able to hit farther with a four iron than you can with a five wood. It's where the ball flies and stops that matters.

It has been reported that more and more players are using the more lofted fairway woods for driving. They find these clubs easier and more accurate to play. Don't think about how far you are *supposed* to be able to hit a shot with any particular club: the point is rather how far *do* you hit it without forcing the shot.

When you're on the tee with your driver, don't force that either. You'll get quite enough distance out of your normal swing if you make it properly. Dis-

CHAPTER 14

tance off the tee is not the name of the game we're playing. Scoring is. Being able to outdrive your competition means nothing. Being able to outscore him means everything.

If you are lucky enough to find a practice range that has a sand trap, practice playing out of it. You can rejoice in the fact that you're in there by choice.

Remember Bobby Locke's comment that he was striking the ball well, but a bit more frequently. The more frequently you strike the ball on the practice range, the less frequently you will strike it on the golf course.

Like riding your stationary bike, practicing golf can only be boring if you let it be. Play each practice shot with as much care and concentration as if it means the match.

We have one friend who, when he has finished practicing through his irons and fairway woods, imagines himself playing a golf course that he can visualize with his eyes shut. He imagines himself driving from the first tee. He knows exactly where he wants to drive the ball. After he hits the shot, he knows, on that familiar hole, where it *did* go. He then analyzes the next shot. Perhaps it is a long par 4 and he has a fairway wood left to hit the green. He goes back to the grassy practice area and plays that shot. If it's long enough and straight enough, he figures he's on the green. Then he resists the temptation to make a 60-foot birdie putt and takes a par. He hasn't three-putted a hole on his imaginary course since we've known him.

STAYING LOOSE AND HAVING FUN

There is an old golfing remark that has amused a lot of people over the years: "Is my friend in the bunker, or is the stinker on the green?"

Much has been written about the "killer instinct" and the true nature of the competitive spirit. Leo Durocher's comment, "Nice guys finish last," has, unfortunately, become a catch phrase of supposed wisdom. When Wellington remarked that the battle of Waterloo had been won on the playing fields of Eton, he wasn't referring to the development of the killer instinct in the young, but to the development of character through sports.

During a 1977 major championship, Charles Coody, who won the 1971 Masters, described one golfer's answer to the competitive drive in saying, "My problem is not with my opponents, it is with myself."

An ideal day of golf includes lovely weather, good companionship and playing close to your best. Sometimes you get one or two of these factors, sometimes all three and, once in a while, none. But the kind of "grand" golfer that the St. Andrews caddy was referring to has enough emotional stability and control of himself and his golf game to take the bad days with the good, because he realizes that he is playing golf for a lifetime and what will live in his memory are the best days, not the worst.

CHAPTER 14

Common sense can help you enjoy your golfing years: guarding against overexposure to the sun, dressing properly for cold and rain, knowing enough to stay away from trees in an electrical storm, taking salt pills if you have been sweating profusely during a match or after a sauna bath.

Many people are on low-salt or salt-free diets. Doubtless their doctors had reasons for prescribing this treatment. However, if your exercise program causes increased loss of body fluids due to sweating, your doctor might well advise judicious use of salt pills to keep your body chemistry in balance.

Let's clear up a couple of points about sweating. No doubt about it, sweating is good for you. It is the body's way of getting rid of excess heat. But don't confuse sweating with weight loss. The number of pounds you lose in a workout or a sauna will be replaced in a matter of hours by what you drink to put the body back in liquid balance.

Golfers in a pressure-packed situation sometimes break out in a light sweat from pure tension. When you are this "pumped up" you might even feel your muscles—in your hands and arms particularly—begin to quiver and jump. Sensing a crisis, your body has given your whole system a jolt of adrenalin, pure energy. If you were a cornered animal facing an enemy, this energy would equip you to either fight or run, just as it was supposed to.

This is great, to be sure, for a cornered animal, but it's tough on a golfer who can't either fight *or* run. Supercharged with new energy, he has to perform a relaxed, precise and highly controlled act.

There isn't too much he can do about it, but just knowing what caused the condition may help. The body wants to explode in a release of energy and will be hard to control. In some cases, depending on the shot to be played, this knowledge may affect club choice: for example, a normal six-iron shot might be hit to the length of a full five iron. When you're feeling this way it may help to do a little deep abdominal breathing as you are lining up the shot, especially if it's a putt.

Those of you who watched the sudden-death playoff in the 1977 PGA Championship may have caught a glimpse of Lanny Wadkins walking down the fairway of one of the extra holes. He carried a club behind his neck and was moving his shoulders as if he were doing the last of our warm-up exercises. Of course he didn't need warming up—what he needed was relief from the tension that was gripping his whole body. This sensation is well known to championship golfers. It is also familiar to millions of men and women at any level of golf play.

SOME WORDS FOR THE WISE

As a doctor, I cannot overemphasize the importance of getting your body into decent condition and keeping it there. While most of you will agree with this advice in theory, you may not act on it for any one of a dozen reasons. Some will put the idea aside as

CHAPTER 14

requiring too rigid a commitment of time and discipline. Others may begin a conditioning program and then drop it because they choose too ambitious a schedule and quickly find themselves exhausted, sore and discouraged.

It doesn't have to be this way. If you begin by doing just the warm-up exercises every day, or every other day, and ease into a more advanced program as time and inclination suggest, you'll soon develop an exercise *habit*. Your body will let you know how much it appreciates and *needs* this activity.

A personal exercise program developed with the aid of this book will help lower your score and your blood pressure, add yards to your drives, years to your life, and create a great new feeling of vitality and satisfaction.

So take it easy, take it a day at a time, and remember that the bad shots you hit yesterday won't count on today's score card.

WEIGHT CONTROL CALORIE COUNTER

EQUIVALENTS USED IN THE FOLLOWING TABLES

$$
\begin{aligned}
1 \text{ quart} &= 4 \text{ cups} \\
1 \text{ cup} &= 8 \text{ fluid ounces} \\
&= \tfrac{1}{2} \text{ pint} \\
&= 16 \text{ tablespoons} \\
2 \text{ tablespoons} &= 1 \text{ fluid ounce} \\
1 \text{ stick butter or margarine} &= \tfrac{1}{2} \text{ cup} \\
&= 16 \text{ pats or squares}
\end{aligned}
$$

Food	Approximate Portion	Calories
Beverages		
Alcoholic, beer (4% alcohol)	2 cups	228
Dessert wines (18.8% alcohol)	½ cup	164
Gin, rum, vodka, whiskey (86 proof)	1 oz.	70
Table wines (12.2% alcohol)	½ cup	100
Carbonated drinks		
Artificially sweetened	12 oz.	0
Club soda	12 oz.	0
Cola drinks, sweetened	12 oz.	137
Fruit-flavored soda	12 oz.	161
Ginger ale	12 oz.	105
Root beer	12 oz.	140

WEIGHT CONTROL CALORIE COUNTER

Food	Approximate Portion	Calories
Coffee, black, unsweetened	1 cup	3
Tea, clear, unsweetened	1 cup	4
Breads, Cereals, Grains and Grain Products		
Biscuits, 2½ in. diameter	1	130
Bran flakes	1 cup	117
Bread, cracked wheat	1 slice	60
Rye	1 slice	55
White	1 slice	60
Whole-wheat	1 slice	55
Corn bread of whole-ground meal	1 serving	100
Cornflakes	1 cup	110
Corn grits, refined, cooked	1 cup	120
Corn meal, yellow	1 cup	360
Crackers, graham	2	55
Soda, 2½ in. square	2	45
Farina	1 cup	105
Flour, soy, full fat	1 cup	460
Wheat, all-purpose	1 cup	400
Wheat, whole	1 cup	390
Macaroni, cooked	1 cup	155
Baked with cheese	1 cup	475
Muffins of refined flour	1	135
Noodles	1 cup	200
Oatmeal, or rolled oats	1 cup	150
Pancakes, buckwheat, 4 in. diam.	4	250
Wheat, refined flour, 4 in. diam.	4	250
Pizza, cheese, ⅛ of 14-in. pie	1 section	180
Popcorn, with oil and salt	2 cups	152
Puffed rice	1 cup	55
Puffed wheat, presweetened	1 cup	105
Rice, brown	1 cup	748
Converted	1 cup	677

WEIGHT CONTROL CALORIE COUNTER

Food	Approximate Portion	Calories
White	1 cup	692
Rice flakes	1 cup	115
Rice, polished	½ cup	132
Rolls, breakfast, sweet	1 large	411
Of refined flour	1	115
Whole-wheat	1	102
Spaghetti with meat sauce	1 cup	285
With tomatoes and cheese	1 cup	210
Spanish rice with meat	1 cup	217
Shredded wheat, biscuit	1	100
Waffles, ½ by 4½ by 5½ in.	1	240
Wheat germ	1 cup	245
Wheat-germ cereal, toasted	1 cup	260
Wheat-meal cereal, unrefined	¼ cup	103
Wheat, unground, cooked, "enriched" (measured before cooking)	¾ cup	275
Dairy Products		
Cows' milk, whole	1 qt.	660
Skim	1 qt.	360
Buttermilk, cultured	1 cup	127
Evaporated milk, undiluted	1 cup	345
Powdered milk, whole	1 cup	515
Skim, instant	1⅓ cups	290
Skim, non-instant	⅔ cup	290
Goat's milk, fresh	1 cup	165
Malted milk (½ cup ice cream)	2 cups	690
Cocoa	1 cup	235
Yogurt, of partially skim milk	1 cup	120
Milk pudding (cornstarch)	1 cup	275
Custard, baked	1 cup	285
Ice cream, commercial	1 cup	300
Ice milk, commercial	1 cup	275
Cream, light, or half-and-half	½ cup	170

**WEIGHT CONTROL
CALORIE COUNTER**

Food	Approximate Portion	Calories
Cream, heavy, or whipping	½ cup	430
Cheese, cottage, creamed	1 cup	240
Uncreamed	1 cup	195
Cheddar, or American	1-in. cube	70
Cheddar, grated	½ cup	226
Cream cheese	1 oz.	105
Processed cheese	1 oz.	105
Roquefort type	1 oz.	105
Swiss	1 oz.	105
Eggs, boiled, poached, or raw	2	150
Scrambled, omelet, or fried	2	220
Yolks only	2	120
Desserts and Sweets		
Apple betty	1 serving	150
Bread pudding with raisins	¾ cup	374
Cake, angel food	1 slice	110
Chocolate cake, fudge icing	1 slice	420
Cupcake with icing	1	160
Fruit cake, 2 by 2 by ½ in.	1 slice	105
Gingerbread, 2-in. cube	1 piece	180
Plain cake, without icing	1 slice	180
Sponge cake, without icing	1 slice	115
Candy, caramels	5	104
Chocolate creams	2	130
Fudge, plain, 1-in. square	2 pieces	370
Hard candies	1 oz.	90
Marshmallows, large	5	98
Milk chocolate	2 oz.	290
Chocolate syrup	2 T.	80
Doughnuts, cake type	1	135
Gelatin, made with water	1 cup	155
Honey, strained	2 T.	120
Ice cream, see		
Dairy products		
Ices, lime, orange, etc.	1 cup	117

Food	Approximate Portion	Calories
Jams, marmalades, preserves	1 T.	55
Jellies	1 T.	50
Molasses, blackstrap	1 T.	45
Cane, refined	1 T.	50
Pie, apple, 1/7 of 9-in. pie	1 slice	330
Cherry	1 slice	340
Custard	1 slice	265
Lemon meringue	1 slice	300
Mince	1 slice	340
Pumpkin	1 slice	265
Sugar, beet or cane	1 T.	50
Brown, firm packed, dark	1 cup	815
Syrup, maple	2 T.	100
Table blends	2 T.	110
Tapioca cream pudding	1 cup	335

Fish and Sea Foods

Food	Approximate Portion	Calories
Clams, steamed or canned	3 oz.	87
Cod, broiled	3½ oz.	170
Codfish cakes, fried	2 small	175
Crab meat, cooked	3 oz.	90
Fish sticks, breaded, fried	5	200
Flounder, baked	3½ oz.	200
Haddock, fried	3 oz.	135
Halibut, broiled	3½ oz.	182
Herring, kippered	1 small	211
Lobster, steamed	½ aver.	92
Mackerel, canned	3 oz.	155
Oysters, raw	½ cup	85
Oyster stew, made with milk	1 cup	200
Salmon, canned	3 oz.	120
Sardines, canned	3 oz.	180
Scallops, breaded, fried	3½ oz.	194
Shad, baked	3 oz.	170
Shrimp, steamed	3 oz.	110

WEIGHT CONTROL CALORIE COUNTER

WEIGHT CONTROL
CALORIE COUNTER

Food	Approximate Portion	Calories
Swordfish, broiled	1 steak	180
Tuna, canned, drained	3 oz.	170
Fruits		
Apple juice, fresh or canned	1 cup	125
Apple vinegar	⅓ cup	14
Apples, raw	1 med.	70
Stewed or canned	1 cup	100
Apricots, canned in syrup	1 cup	220
Dried, uncooked	½ cup	220
Fresh	3 med.	55
Nectar, or juice	1 cup	140
Avocado	½ large	185
Banana	1 med.	85
Blackberries, fresh	1 cup	85
Blueberries, canned	1 cup	245
Cantaloupe	½ med.	40
Cherries, canned, pitted	1 cup	100
Fresh, raw	1 cup	65
Cranberry sauce, sweetened	1 cup	530
Dates, dried	1 cup	505
Figs, dried, large, 2 in. by 1 in.	2	120
Fresh, raw	3 med.	90
Stewed or canned, with syrup	3	130
Fruit cocktail, canned	1 cup	195
Grapefruit, canned sections	1 cup	170
Grapefruit, fresh, 5 in. diam.	½	50
Grapefruit juice	1 cup	100
Grapes, American, as Concord	1 cup	70
European, as Muscat, Tokay	1 cup	100
Grape juice, bottled	1 cup	160
Lemon juice, fresh	½ cup	30

WEIGHT CONTROL CALORIE COUNTER

Food	Approximate Portion	Calories
Lemonade concentrate, frozen	6 oz. can	430
Limeade concentrate, frozen	6 oz. can	405
Olives, green, canned, large	10	72
Ripe, canned, large	10	105
Oranges, fresh 3 in. diam.	1 med.	60
Frozen concentrate	6 oz. can	330
Papaya, fresh	½ med.	75
Peaches, canned, sliced	1 cup	200
Fresh, raw	1 med.	35
Pears, canned, sweetened	1 cup	195
Raw, 3 in. by 2½ in.	1 med.	100
Persimmons, Japanese	1 med.	75
Pineapple, canned sliced	1 large slice	95
Crushed	1 cup	205
Raw, diced	1 cup	75
Pineapple juice, canned	1 cup	120
Plums, canned in syrup	1 cup	185
Raw, 2 in. diam.	1	30
Prunes, cooked	1 cup	300
Prune juice, canned	1 cup	170
Raisins, dried	½ cup	230
Raspberries, frozen	½ cup	100
Raw, red	¾ cup	57
Rhubarb, cooked, sweetened	1 cup	385
Strawberries, frozen	1 cup	242
Raw	1 cup	54
Tangerines, fresh	1 med.	40
Watermelon, 4 in. by 8 in.	1 wedge	120
Meat and Poultry, cooked		
Bacon, crisp, drained	2 slices	95
Beef, chuck, pot-roasted	3 oz.	245
Hamburger, commercial	3 oz.	245
Ground lean	3 oz.	185
Roast beef, oven-cooked	3 oz.	390
Steak, lean, as round	3 oz.	220

WEIGHT CONTROL CALORIE COUNTER

Food	Approximate Portion	Calories
Corned beef	3 oz.	185
Corned beef hash, canned	3 oz.	120
Dried or chipped	2 oz.	115
Pot-pie, 4½ in. diam.	1 pie	460
Stew, with vegetables	1 cup	185
Chicken, broiled	3 oz.	185
Fried, breast or leg and thigh	3 oz.	245
Roasted	3½ oz.	290
Chicken livers, fried	3 med.	140
Duck, domestic	3½ oz.	370
Lamb, chop, broiled	4 oz.	480
Leg, roasted	3 oz.	314
Shoulder, braised	3 oz.	285
Pork, chop, 1 thick	3½ oz.	260
Ham, cured, pan-broiled	3 oz.	290
Ham, as luncheon meat	2 oz.	170
Ham, canned, spiced	2 oz.	165
Pork roast	3 oz.	310
Pork sausage, bulk	3½ oz.	475
Turkey, roasted	3½ oz.	265
Veal, cutlet, broiled	3 oz.	185
Roast	3 oz.	305
Meats—Variety		
Brains, beef, calf, pork, sheep	3½ oz.	125
Chili con carne with beans	1 cup	325
Without beans	1 cup	510
Heart, braised	3 oz.	160
Kidney, braised	3½ oz.	230
Liver, beef, sauteed with oil	3½ oz.	230
Calf, 1 large slice	3½ oz.	261
Lamb, 2 slices	3½ oz.	260
Pork, 2 slices	3½ oz.	241
Sausages, bologna	2 slices, ⅛ by 4 in.	124

WEIGHT CONTROL CALORIE COUNTER

Food	Approximate Portion	Calories
Frankfurter	2, ¾ by 7 in.	246
Liverwurst	2 oz.	132
Sweetbreads, calf, braised	3½ oz.	170
Tongue, beef	3 oz.	205
Nuts, Nut Products and Seeds		
Almonds, dried	½ cup	425
Roasted and salted	½ cup	439
Brazil nuts, unsalted	½ cup	457
Cashews, unsalted	½ cup	392
Coconut, shredded, sweetened	½ cup	274
Peanut butter, commercial	⅓ cup	300
Natural	⅓ cup	284
Peanuts, roasted	⅓ cup	290
Pecans, raw, halves	½ cup	343
Sesame seeds, dry	½ cup	280
Sunflower seeds	½ cup	280
Walnuts, English, raw	½ cup	325
Oils, Fats and Shortenings		
Butter	1 T.	100
Hydrogenated cooking fat	½ cup	665
Lard	½ cup	992
Margarine	1 T.	100
Mayonnaise	1 T.	110
Oils		
Corn, soy, peanut, cottonseed	1 T.	125
Olive	1 T.	125
Safflower, sunflower seed, walnut	1 T.	125
Salad dressing		
French	1 T.	60
Thousand Island	1 T.	75
Salt pork	2 oz.	470

WEIGHT CONTROL CALORIE COUNTER

Food	Approximate Portion	Calories
Soups, Canned and Diluted		
(No data available on soups made at home.)		
Bean soups	1 cup	190
Beef and vegetable	1 cup	100
Bouillon, broth, consommé	1 cup	24
Chicken or turkey	1 cup	75
Clam chowder, without milk	1 cup	85
Cream soups (asparagus, celery, etc.)	1 cup	200
Noodle, rice, barley soups	1 cup	115
Split-pea soup	1 cup	147
Tomato soup, diluted with milk	1 cup	175
Vegetable (vegetarian)	1 cup	80
Vegetables		
Artichoke, globe	1 large	8–44
Asparagus, green	6 spears	18
Beans, green snap	1 cup	25
Lima, green	1 cup	140
Lima, dry, cooked	1 cup	260
Navy, baked with pork	¾ cup	250
Red kidney, canned	1 cup	230
Bean sprouts, uncooked	1 cup	17
Beet greens, steamed	1 cup	27
Beetroots, boiled	1 cup	68
Broccoli, steamed	1 cup	45
Brussels sprouts, steamed	1 cup	60
Cabbage, as coleslaw, with mayonnaise	1 cup	140
Sauerkraut, canned	1 cup	32
Steamed cabbage	1 cup	40
Carrots, cooked, diced	1 cup	45
Raw, grated	1 cup	45
Strips, from raw	1 med.	20
Cauliflower, steamed	1 cup	30

WEIGHT CONTROL CALORIE COUNTER

Food	Approximate Portion	Calories
Celery, cooked, diced	1 cup	20
Stalk, raw	1 large	5
Chard, steamed, leaves and stalks	1 cup	30
Collards, steamed leaves	1 cup	51
Corn, steamed	1 ear	92
Cooked or canned	1 cup	170
Cucumbers, ⅛-in. slices	6	6
Dandelion greens, steamed	1 cup	80
Eggplant, steamed	1 cup	30
Endive (escarole)	2 oz.	10
Kale, steamed	1 cup	45
Kohlrabi, raw, sliced	1 cup	40
Lambs'-quarters, steamed	1 cup	48
Lentils	1 cup	212
Lettuce, loose leaf, green	¼ head	14
Iceberg	¼ head	13
Mushrooms, cooked or canned	½ cup	12
Okra, diced, steamed	1⅓ cups	32
Onions, mature, cooked	1 cup	80
Raw, green	6 small	22
Parsley, chopped, raw	2 T.	2
Parsnips, steamed	1 cup	95
Peas, green, canned	1 cup	68
Fresh, steamed	1 cup	70
Frozen, heated	1 cup	68
Split, cooked	½ cup	115
With carrots, frozen, heated	1 cup	53
Peppers, pimientos, canned	1 pod	10
Raw, green, sweet	1 large	25
Stuffed with beef and crumbs	1 med.	255
Potatoes, baked	1 med.	100
French-fried	10 pieces	155
Mashed with milk and butter	1 cup	230
Pan-fried	¾ cup	268

Food	Approximate Portion	Calories
Scalloped with cheese	¾ cup	145
Steamed before peeling	1 med.	80
Potato chips	10	110
Radishes, raw	5 small	10
Rutabagas, diced	⅔ cup	32
Soybeans, unseasoned	1 cup	260
Spinach, steamed	1 cup	26
Squash, summer	1 cup	35
Winter, mashed	1 cup	95
Sweet potatoes, baked	1 med.	155
Candied	1 med.	235
Tomatoes, canned whole	1 cup	50
Raw, 2 in. by 2½ in.	1 med.	30
Tomato juice, canned	1 cup	50
Tomato catsup	1 T.	15
Turnip greens, steamed	1 cup	45
Turnips, steamed, sliced	1 cup	40
Watercress, leaves and stems, raw	1 cup	9